ADVANCE PRAISE FOR *RADIAL ACCESS FOR NEUROINTERVENTION*

"The book is the first of its kind describing a complete & detailed description of Cerebrovascular procedures performed via transradial access. Compiled by world experts in Neuro intervention & detailing how these procedures should be done & nuances associated with this approach. The book is revolutionary & ushers a new era of a set of procedures done via transradial approach which promises to increase patient satisfaction, decrease unwanted complications, reduces cost, & improve outcome. This book is a must to every neurointerventionalist."

—David Hasan, MD, Professor of Neurosurgery,
Otolaryngology, & Biomedical Engineering

"This book focusing on Radial Access for Neurointervention reflects the change in the current mindset on arterial access, and not a moment too soon. The chapters do a great job reviewing the concepts and practice of radial access with great tips and tricks with a mature pragmatic perspective. Fellows and attendings alike will benefit from the knowledge and experiences shared in this book."

—Ameer E. Hassan, Professor of Neurology & Radiology
UTRGV, Head of Neuroscience Department, Valley Baptist Medical Center

RADIAL ACCESS FOR NEUROINTERVENTION

Edited by

Pascal M. Jabbour

The Angela and Richard T. Clark Distinguished
Professor of Neurological Surgery
Division Chief of Neurovascular Surgery
and Endovascular Neurosurgery
Thomas Jefferson University Hospital

and

Eric C. Peterson

Associate Professor of Neurological Surgery
Chief of Endovascular Neurosurgery
University of Miami MILLER School of Medicine
Jackson Memorial Hospital

OXFORD
UNIVERSITY PRESS

OXFORD
UNIVERSITY PRESS

Oxford University Press is a department of the University of Oxford. It furthers
the University's objective of excellence in research, scholarship, and education
by publishing worldwide. Oxford is a registered trade mark of Oxford University
Press in the UK and certain other countries.

Published in the United States of America by Oxford University Press
198 Madison Avenue, New York, NY 10016, United States of America.

Library of Congress Cataloging-in-Publication Data
Names: Pascal M. Jabbour, Eric C. Peterson, editors.
Title: Radial access for neurointervention / Pascal M. Jabbour and Eric C. Peterson.
Description: New York, NY : Oxford University Press, [2021] |
Includes bibliographical references and index.
Identifiers: LCCN 2020055997 (print) | LCCN 2020055998 (ebook) |
ISBN 9780197524176 (hardback) | ISBN 9780197524190 (epub) |
ISBN 9780197524213 (digital-online)
Subjects: MESH: Cerebrovascular Disorders—surgery | Neurosurgical Procedures—methods |
Radial Artery—surgery | Catheterization, Peripheral—methods
Classification: LCC RD593 (print) | LCC RD593 (ebook) |
NLM WL 355 | DDC 617.4/8—dc23
LC record available at https://lccn.loc.gov/2020055997
LC ebook record available at https://lccn.loc.gov/2020055998

DOI: 10.1093/med/9780197524176.001.0001

3 5 7 9 8 6 4 2

Printed by Integrated Books International, United States of America

We want to dedicate this book to our patients, they inspire us every day with their courage.

Contents

Contributors

Fadi Al Saiegh, MD
Neurological Surgery
Thomas Jefferson University
Philadelphia, PA, USA

Marie-Christine Brunet, MD, FRCSC
Neurosurgeon
Department of Neurology and
    Neurosurgery
Montreal Neurologic Institute
Montréal, QC, Canada

Stephanie H. Chen, MD
Physician
Department of Neurosurgery
University of Miami
Miami, FL, USA

Karim Hafazalla, MD
Resident Neurosurgery
Thomas Jefferson University Hospital
Philadelphia, PA, USA

Pascal M. Jabbour, MD
The Angela and Richard T. Clark
    Distinguished Professor of
    Neurological Surgery Division
    Chief of Neurovascular Surgery and
    Endovascular Neurosurgery
Thomas Jefferson University
    Hospital
Philadelphia, PA, USA

Omaditya Khanna, MD
Resident Neurosurgery
Thomas Jefferson University
    Hospital
Philadelphia, PA, USA

Jonathon Lebovitz, MD
Neurosurgeon
Neurosurgery
Danbury Hospital
Danbury, CT, USA

Evan Luther, MD
Resident Physician
Neurological Surgery
University of Miami Miller School of
   Medicine
Miami, FL, USA

Nikolaos Mouchtouris, MD
Resident Physician
Neurosurgery
Thomas Jefferson University
Philadelphia, PA, USA

Eric C. Peterson, MD
Associate Professor of Neurological
   Surgery/Chief of Endovascular
   Neurosurgery
Neurological Surgery
University of Miami/Jackson Memorial
   Hospital
Miami, FL, USA

Kalyan Sajja, MD
Interventional Neurologist
Life Neurovascular Institute
Life Hospital
Guntur, AP, India

Brian Snelling, MD
Chief of Cerebrovascular Neurosurgery
Neurological Surgery
Marcus Neuroscience Institute
Boca Raton, FL, USA

Christopher Storey, MD, PhD
Neurosurgeon
Nashville Neurosurgery Associates
Nashville, TN, USA

Samir Sur, MD
Assistant Professor
Department of Neurosurgery
Georgetown University School of
   Medicine
Washington, DC, USA

Ahmad Sweid, MD
Postdoctoral Research Fellow
Neurological Surgery
Thomas Jefferson University
Philadelphia, PA, USA

CHAPTER 1

The Rationale for Radial Artery Access in Neurointerventional Surgery

SAMIR SUR, STEPHANIE H. CHEN,
PASCAL M. JABBOUR, AND ERIC C. PETERSON

INTRODUCTION

Endovascular techniques have revolutionized surgery for vascular disease. Most arterial structures—whether in the chest, brain, or abdomen—reside deep in the body, and exposing them surgically is a major undertaking. Whether it is a craniotomy, medial sternotomy, or abdominal exposure, a significant part of the risk of the surgery is just accessing the blood vessels. Transfemoral endovascular surgery was initially pioneered in interventional cardiology. Because the coronary vessels are large and straight, it was relatively straightforward to develop catheter systems to access them. As catheter systems became more sophisticated, endovascular surgery expanded from cardiac applications to neurointerventional and peripheral interventional fields. Both are now dominated by endovascular techniques due to their minimal invasiveness. The common femoral artery has been the primary access site for neuroendovascular angiography and interventions since the emergence of the field, owing to its large caliber and compressible location superficial to the head of the femur.[1]

However, less invasive does not mean noninvasive. Despite progress in closure devices as well as access catheter and sheath design, access-site complications remain a clinically important risk of transfemoral endovascular surgery.[2] The potential space present in the proximal lower extremity allows for large hematomas or the formation of pseudo-aneurysms, which can be associated with significant morbidity. In addition, inadvertent arterial puncture above the inguinal ligament threatens the rare but potentially catastrophic retroperitoneal hematoma.[2,3]

Last, the common femoral artery is an end artery, and thrombosis results in acute limb-threatening ischemia. Regardless of careful access and closure technique, these anatomical features are fixed. Thus, in the late 1980s, interventional cardiologists first described a transradial approach (TRA) for percutaneous coronary angiography as a means of reducing the significant access-site bleeding complications that accompanied the increasing use of anticoagulants and large-bore catheter systems.[4]

The radial artery has two principal anatomical advantages as an access site as compared to the femoral artery. First, the radial artery courses superficially in the forearm and is easily compressed against the distal radius. There is very little potential space in the distal forearm; therefore, hematoma formation is limited, easily identified, and controlled. Second, as opposed to the common femoral artery, the robust collateral circulation to the hand via the palmar arch and interosseous branches renders inadvertent radial artery occlusion clinically silent (Figure 1.1).[5]

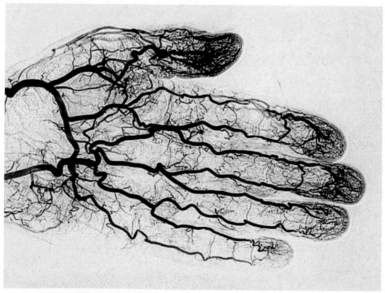

FIGURE 1.1 *Hand collaterals. Note the extensive and redundant arterial supply to the hand.*

WHY RADIAL: SAFETY

Over the ensuing decades, a mountain of prospective, randomized evidence has confirmed that the anatomic advantages of TRA results in a dramatic reduction in access-site complications and even mortality when compared to the transfemoral approach (TFA). In 2018, the American Heart Association offered an update to its guidelines on angiography and intervention in acute coronary syndrome (ACS) and concluded, "TRA should be considered the default strategy in the invasive management of patients with ACS."[6]

Multiple large-scale trials comparing TRA to TFA have been performed. In the STEMI-RADIAL trial of 707 patients, major access-site bleeding and complication rate was 7.2% in the femoral cohort and 1.4% in the radial cohort.[7] In the RIFLE-STEACS trial with 1000 patients, major access-site complications again were found to be 6.8% in the femoral group and 2.6% in the radial group.[8] Similarly, the rate of major access-site complications from the ESCAPE and SWIFT-PRIME trials, femoral-only trials of mechanical thrombectomy, were also approximately 7%.[9,10] This suggests good external validity from the interventional cardiology access-site trials to the neurointerventional population (see Table 1.1).

Even larger randomized trials have been subsequently performed, including the 7021-patient RIVAL trial[11] and the 8404-patient MATRIX trial,[12] both of which found significant decreases in access-site complications with TRA as compared to TFA. In addition to their large size, these trials offered two additional insights. First, the MATRIX trial

TABLE 1.1 Summary of Major Interventional Cardiology Trials Comparing Transradial and Transfemoral Access

Trial Name	No. of Patients	Primary Endpoint (TR vs. TF)	Major Bleeding (TR vs. TF)	Access-Site Complications (TR vs. TF)	All-Cause Mortality (TR vs. TF)
RIVAL[11]	7021	3.7% vs. 4.0%; $p = 0.50$	0.7% vs. 0.9%; $p = 0.23$	1.4% vs. 3.7%; $p < 0.0001$	1.3% vs. 1.5%; $p = 0.47$
MATRIX[12]	8404	8.8% vs. 10.3%; $p = 0.03072$	1.6% vs. 2.3%; $p = 0.013$	0.1% vs. 0.4%; $p = 0.0115$	1.6% vs. 2.2%; $p = 0.045$
RIFLE-STEACS[8]	1001	13.6% vs. 21.0%; $p = 0.003$	2.6% vs. 6.8%; $p = 0.002$	N/A	5.2% vs. 9.2%; $p = 0.020$
STEMI-RADIAL[7]	707	1.4% vs. 7.2%; $p = 0.0001$	1.4% vs. 7.2%; $p = 0.0001$	0.3% vs. 0.8%; $p = 0.62$	2.3% vs. 3.1%; $p = 0.64$

Note that specific definitions for various endpoints differ among the trials. Access-site complications have generally been defined as those requiring intervention (transfusion, repair, or active surveillance) or hematoma that met predetermined size criteria. Refer to individual trial manuscripts for specific criteria. Abbreviations: TR, transradial; TF, transfemoral.

was adequately powered to discover a mortality benefit with TRA simply from avoiding the femoral artery as an access site (1.6% vs. 2.2%, $p = 0.045$).[12] Second, the RIVAL trial showed a much smaller femoral complication rate than other trials (3.7%), but this was still over 3 times that of the TRA group (1.4%, HR 0.37, 95% CI 0.27–0.52, $p < 0.001$).[11] This again supports the notion that no matter how careful you are with femoral access and closure, you cannot change the anatomic limitations of the femoral artery as an access site discussed earlier, and that TRA consistently takes advantage of those anatomical differences to offer a safe access alternative. This is demonstrated in Figure 1.2, where a meta-analysis of randomized controlled trials comparing TRA and TFA illustrates the consistent safety advantage of TRA.

The neurointerventional field is significantly smaller than that of interventional cardiology, and large randomized controlled trials with 8000 patients will unlikely ever be achieved for neurointervention. However, given the similarities between the two fields as they relate to access (similar bore catheters, need for full heparinization, and use of dual antiplatelet agents), as well as the identical arterial sites (radial and femoral arteries), it seems unlikely that the significant safety advantages of TRA for interventional cardiology would not be true in neurointervention. Indeed, already there are investigations in the neurointerventional literature that as expected show a favorable safety profile of TRA over TFA. Catapano et al. retrospectively evaluated over 1000 patients in their center and showed a complication rate for TFA of 7% as opposed to 2% for TRA—almost identical to the cardiac trials.[13] In multiple other reported series of transradial access for neuroendovascular procedures, access-site complication rates have been low, and these early data offer support for decreased morbidity compared to TFA in this population as well.[14–21]

WHY RADIAL: ANATOMICAL CONSIDERATIONS

Safety advantages of TRA aside, there are a multitude of clinical scenarios where TFA is a suboptimal access site and being facile at TRA is critical. The simplest is severe aorto-femoral occlusive disease, or Leriche syndrome. In this situation, TFA is simply not possible. Ribo et al. evaluated a consecutive cohort of 136 stroke patients undergoing mechanical thrombectomy and found that in 5% catheterization of the carotid artery was unable to be achieved.[22] In these scenarios, simply converting to TRA allows the operator to bypass the aorto-femoral occlusive disease and access the great vessels in short order.

The second clinical scenario where the anatomy favors TRA is in severe arch tortuosity or bovine arch configurations. Both result in a very challenging vector for the catheters to be navigated in TFA, and both are easier to navigate from the arm. Kaesmacher et al. evaluated over 600 patients undergoing mechanical thrombectomy via the femoral approach and found that in over one-third of the reperfusion failures the reason for failure was inability to

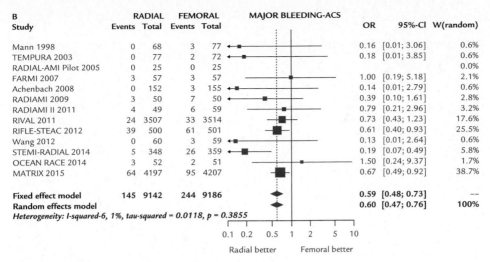

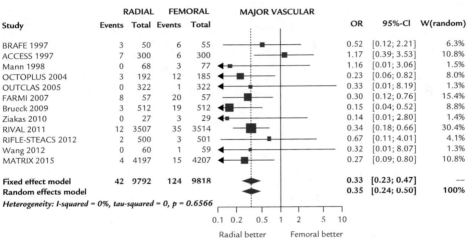

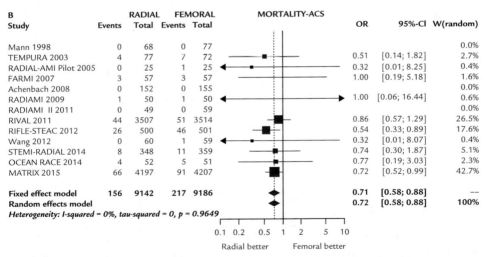

FIGURE 1.2 *Meta-analysis of cardiac randomized controlled trials comparing transradial approach to transfemoral approach.*

Source: Mason PJ, Shah B, Tamis-Holland JE, Bittl JA, Cohen MG, Safirstein J, Drachman DE, Valle JA, Rhodes D, Gilchrist IC. An update on radial artery access and best practices for transradial coronary angiography and intervention in acute coronary syndrome: a scientific statement from the American Heart Association. *Circ Cardiovasc Interv.* 2018;11(9):e000035.

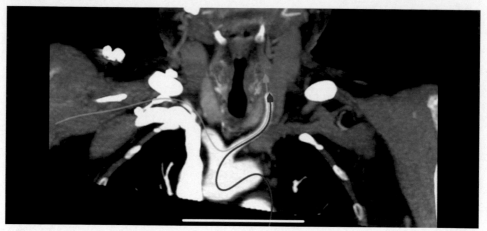

FIGURE 1.3 *Bovine configuration arch demonstrating the more favorable angle of navigation from the transradial approach (green arrow) versus the transfemoral approach (purple arrow).*

catheterize the target vessel.[23] Even in the patients where catheterization was eventually able to be achieved, Ribo et al. found that the chances of a good outcome in the slowest quartile dropped to 1 in 10—even when time to revascularization was controlled for.[22] As shown in Figure 1.3, the angle for TRA in these difficult arch patients is more favorable than for TFA.

The third clinical scenario that favors TRA over TFA is in posterior circulation interventions.[24] Particularly for right vertebral artery (VA) interventions, but also for left vertebral, the access to the VA from the ipsilateral arm is much more straightforward than from the femoral artery. With the introduction of the snuffbox or distal radial technique (discussed in detail in Chapter 3), left radial access to the left VA is straightforward as the left hand can be positioned in the midline.

WHY RADIAL: PATIENT PREFERENCE

Interestingly, although the initial impetus for TRA was safety, extensive data support a strong patient preference for TRA over TFA.[25-27] As we tell our fellows: "The femoral access site is not in the leg—it's in the groin." Even without a complication, the femoral access site is an unpleasant location to be stuck, and it is often sore after a procedure. Furthermore, the 2 to 6 hours of immobilization after TFA is universally despised by patients. Here, the transradial technique is again superior to the traditional TFA. Closure of the radial arteriotomy is accomplished with direct compression of the puncture site, and this is easily performed with manual compression or application of a bracelet which can be inflated to provide compression to achieve patent hemostasis ("TR Band," Terumo, Somerset, NJ). Thus, for TRA cases, patients are able to ambulate immediately and have relatively full use of the affected upper extremity while the TR Band is in place (typically 30 minutes to 1 hour after the conclusion of the procedure).

Unsurprisingly, this benefit is both preferred by patients and offers an additional benefit of cost reduction (in terms of postprocedural nursing requirements and hospital stay) beyond those achieved by access-site morbidity reduction.[14,18,28] Again, while specific cost analysis in patients undergoing neurointerventional procedures remains to be reported on a large scale, in this context, extrapolated data in combination with rationality and common sense should determine best practice.

REFERENCES

1. Richling B. History of endovascular surgery: personal accounts of the evolution. *Neurosurgery.* 2006;59:S30–S38;discussion S3–13.

2. Sreeram S et al. Retroperitoneal hematoma following femoral arterial catheterization: a serious and often fatal complication. *Am Surg.* 1993;59:94–98.

3. Chan YC, Morales JP, Reidy JF, Taylor, PR. Management of spontaneous and iatrogenic retroperitoneal haemorrhage: conservative management, endovascular intervention or open surgery? *Int J Clin Pract.* 2008;62:1604–1613.

4. Kiemeneij F. The history and evolution of transradial coronary interventions. In: *Transradial Approach for Percutaneous Interventions.* xx; 2017:3–7. doi:10.1007/978-94-017-7350-8_1.

5. Stella PR et al. Incidence and outcome of radial artery occlusion following transradial artery coronary angioplasty. *Cathet Cardiovasc Diagn.* 1997;40:156–158.

6. Mason PJ et al. An update on radial artery access and best practices for transradial coronary angiography and intervention in acute coronary syndrome: a scientific statement from the American Heart Association. *Circ Cardiovasc Interv.* 2018;11:e000035.

7. Bernat I et al. ST-segment elevation myocardial infarction treated by radial or femoral approach in a multicenter randomized clinical trial: the STEMI-RADIAL trial. *J Am Coll Cardiol.* 2014;63:964–972.

8. Romagnoli E et al. Radial versus femoral randomized investigation in ST-segment elevation acute coronary syndrome: the RIFLE-STEACS (Radial Versus Femoral Randomized Investigation in ST-Elevation Acute Coronary Syndrome) study. *J Am Coll Cardiol.* 2012;60:2481–2489.

9. Goyal M et al. Randomized assessment of rapid endovascular treatment of ischemic stroke. *N Engl J Med.* 2015;372:1019–1030.

10. Saver JL et al. Stent-retriever thrombectomy after intravenous t-PA versus t-PA alone in stroke. *N Engl J Med.* 2015;372:2285–2295.

11. Jolly SS et al. Radial versus femoral access for coronary angiography and intervention in patients with acute coronary syndromes (RIVAL): a randomised, parallel group, multicentre trial. *Lancet.* 2011;377:1409–1420.

12. Valgimigli M et al. Radial versus femoral access in patients with acute coronary syndromes undergoing invasive management: a randomised multicentre trial. *Lancet.* 2015;385:2465–2476.

13. Catapano JS, Fredrickson VL, Fujii T et al. Complications of femoral versus radial access in neuroendovascular procedures with propensity adjustment. *J Neurointerv Surg.* 2020;12:611–615. doi:10.1136/neurintsurg-2019-015569.

14. Snelling BM et al. Transradial cerebral angiography: techniques and outcomes. *J Neurointerv Surg.* 2018;10:874–881.

15. Chen SH, Snelling BM, Shah SS et al. Transradial approach for flow diversion treatment of cerebral aneurysms: a multicenter study. *J Neurointerv Surg.* 2019;11:796–800. doi:10.1136/neurintsurg-2018-014620.

16. Chen SH, Snelling BM, Sur S et al. Transradial versus transfemoral access for anterior circulation mechanical thrombectomy: comparison of technical and clinical outcomes. *J Neurointerv Surg.* 2019;11:874–878. doi:10.1136/neurintsurg-2018-014485.

17. Snelling BM et al. Transradial approach for complex anterior and posterior circulation interventions: technical nuances and feasibility of using current devices. *Oper Neurosurg (Hagerstown).* 2019;17(3):293–302. doi:10.1093/ons/opy352.

18. Khanna O et al. Radial artery catheterization for neuroendovascular procedures: clinical outcomes and patient satisfaction measures. *Stroke.* 2019;50:2587–2590.

19. Zussman BM et al. A prospective study of the transradial approach for diagnostic cerebral arteriography. *J Neurointerv Surg.* 2019;11:1045–1049.

20. Stone JG, Zussman BM, Tonetti DA et al. Transradial versus transfemoral approaches for diagnostic cerebral angiography: a prospective, single-center, non-inferiority comparative effectiveness study. *J Neurointerv Surg.* 2020;12(10):993–998. doi:10.1136/neurintsurg-2019-015642.

21. Almallouhi E et al. Fast-track incorporation of the transradial approach in endovascular neurointervention. *J Neurointerv Surg.* 2020;12:176–180.

22. Ribo M et al. Difficult catheter access to the occluded vessel during endovascular treatment of acute ischemic stroke is associated with worse clinical outcome. *J Neurointerv Surg.* 2013;5:i70–i73.

23. Kaesmacher J et al. Reasons for reperfusion failures in stent-retriever-based thrombectomy: registry analysis and proposal of a classification system. *J Neuroradiol.* 2018;39:1848–1853.

24. Maud A et al. Transradial access results in faster skin puncture to reperfusion time than transfemoral access in posterior circulation mechanical thrombectomy. *J Vasc Interv Neurol.* 2019;10:53–57.

25. Kok MM et al. Patient preference for radial versus femoral vascular access for elective coronary procedures: the PREVAS study. *Catheter Cardiovasc Interv.* 2018;91:17–24.

26. Liu LB et al. Patient experience and preference in transradial versus transfemoral access during transarterial radioembolization: a randomized single-center trial. *J Vasc Interv Radiol.* 2019;30:414–420.

27. Satti SR, Vance AZ, Golwala SN, Eden T. Patient preference for transradial access over transfemoral access for cerebrovascular procedures. *J Vasc Interv Neurol.* 2017;9:1–5.

28. Cooper CJ et al. Effect of transradial access on quality of life and cost of cardiac catheterization: a randomized comparison. *Am Heart J.* 1999;138:430–436.

CHAPTER 2

Transradial Access Techniques

EVAN LUTHER, STEPHANIE H. CHEN, PASCAL M. JABBOUR, AND ERIC C. PETERSON

INTRODUCTION

Numerous studies have demonstrated a significant benefit with the transradial approach (TRA) as compared to the traditional transfemoral approach (TFA) in decreasing access-site complications, reducing cost, and improving patient experience. For this reason, the American Heart Association recommends a "radial first" strategy for acute coronary syndrome. With a growing body of evidence supporting transradial neurointerventional procedures, the neurointerventional community will likely follow. In this chapter, we describe the basic technique for setting up and performing radial access.

ROOM SET-UP AND POSITIONING FOR STANDARD RIGHT TRANSRADIAL ACCESS

The vast majority of TRA for cerebral angiography and interventions is performed via the right radial artery. In the preoperative area, a thin film of 2.5% lidocaine/prilocaine topical cream is applied to the wrist and then covered with an adhesive dressing to protect the local anesthetic from inadvertent removal (Figure 2.1). The topical lidocaine

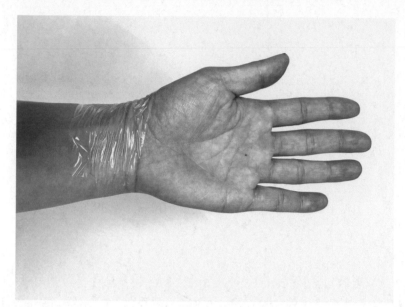

FIGURE 2.1 *Preoperative preparation of the wrist where an adhesive dressing is placed over a thin film of 2.5% lidocaine/prilocaine topical cream that is applied to the wrist.*

should be applied to both the proximal and distal (snuffbox) skin sites. After 30 minutes, the dressing is removed, and the patient is brought to the angiography suite.[1,2] A pulse oximeter is placed on the ipsilateral thumb to monitor hand perfusion, and the patient is placed supine on the angiography table. Padding is placed underneath the entire length of the arm, terminating just distal to the fingertips so that the wrist remains level with the hip, thus ensuring that the catheter is in a position similar to that seen in the TFA (Figure 2.2).[1,4]

The arm is placed supine as close to the hip as possible.[2] Full supination of the hand is not necessary, and this is often uncomfortable for patients, particularly elderly patients. We simply use a piece of tape to hold the hand in position and another piece of tape to gently retract the thenar eminence of the thumb to allow access to the proximal radial artery just above the wrist crease (Figures 2.3 and 2.4). Other options include commercial braces to assist in the hand position.

Critical to radial access is the placement of a support board inferior to the hand next to the knee (red arrow, Figure 2.2). The reason for this is that unlike femoral access where the catheters can rest on the legs, radial access is a more lateral access site, resulting in the catheters falling down off the legs (Figure 2.5) unless a place for them to rest is provided. There are many ways to achieve this, but the goal is a completely flat surface for the proximal portion of the catheters to rest so the operator does not have to do anything different

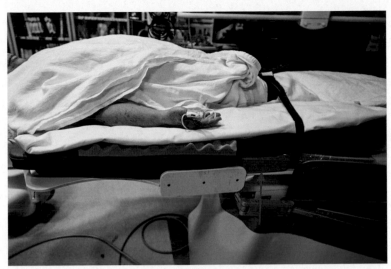

FIGURE 2.2 *Positioning of the hand on sufficient padding underneath the entire length of the arm and distal to the hand (red arrow), ensuring that the working space is level with the hip to prevent any catheters from falling off the table.*

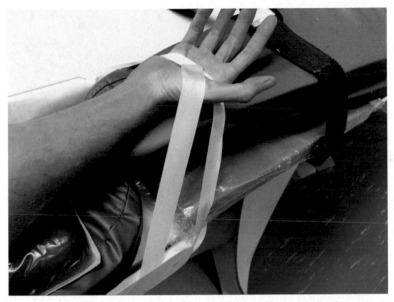

FIGURE 2.3 *Tape is used to hold the hand in position and gently retract the thenar eminence of the thumb to allow access to the proximal radial artery 1–2 cm above the wrist crease (black arrow).*

than a femoral case once access is obtained. Figure 2.2 shows our preferred set-up, and Figure 2.6 shows the result once prepped. Note the completely flat surface to avoid having to curve the catheters back to the legs or awkward bending of the operator to reach over the legs.

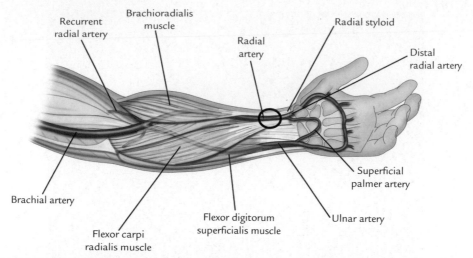

FIGURE 2.4 *Illustration of radial artery anatomy. Access should be obtained 1–2 cm above the wrist crease below the brachioradialis tendon (black circle).*

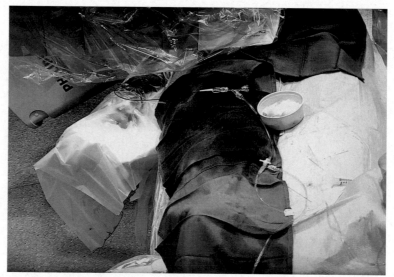

FIGURE 2.5 *An example of poor arm positioning where the arm is too lateral and there is insufficient padding distal to the hand, resulting in bending of catheters or risk of catheters falling off the table.*

Once the patient is positioned, the anteroposterior (AP) plane is brought into position in the "head position" in the midline. The elbow is brought into the field. In the event that patient anatomy precludes visualization of the elbow with the AP plane in the midline, the table is rotated clockwise 5–10 degrees to bring the elbow into view (Figure 2.7).

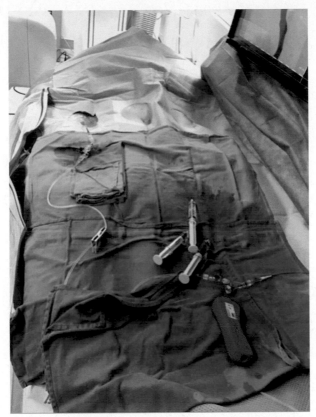

FIGURE 2.6 *An example of appropriate radial set-up with a completely flat surface.*

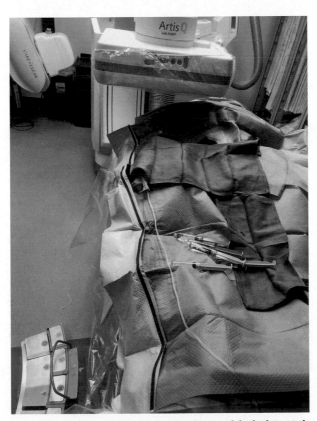

FIGURE 2.7 *In patients with large body habitus, angulation of the bed 5–10 degrees may be necessary to capture the brachial bifurcation with the anteroposterior plane head side.*

ROOM SET-UP AND POSITIONING FOR LEFT TRANSRADIAL ACCESS

Although left TRA is common in cardiology due to the anatomically favorable position of the left subclavian origin for coronary artery access, it is relatively rare in neuroangiography because of the ease of catheterizing all of the great vessels from the right radial approach.[3,6,7] In the event that left transradial access is needed (usually for posterior circulation interventions when right vertebral artery is hypoplastic), the left arm is not positioned next to the patient.[2,3] Instead, the hand is pulled through the left femoral opening in the drape and placed on the patient's abdomen in the midline with the elbow bent slightly (Figure 2.8).[3] This allows the operator to access the left radial artery from the right side of the patient and to avoid uncomfortable bending over the patient to reach the left hand during the intervention.

Given the inherent difficulty associated with supinating the left hand with the arm in this position, most operators prefer using the left anatomic snuffbox for access.[7,8] Thus, the wrist and hand are again left in a more anatomically neutral position with the hand slightly pronated and deviated in the ulnar direction to again expose the anatomical snuffbox.[2,5]

ACCESS TECHNIQUE

Anatomic Landmarks

For standard TRA, the radial artery is typically accessed 1–2 cm proximal to the wrist crease (black circle, Figure 2.4). If spasm is encountered, the operator can move more

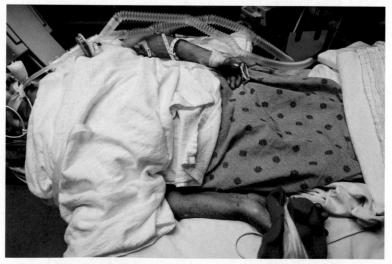

FIGURE 2.8 *Left distal transradial access hand positioning wherein the arm is draped across the patient's abdomen to the midline with the elbow bent slightly.*

proximally to access the radial artery proximal to the spasm. Great care should be made to not puncture too proximally, when the radial artery has not exited from under the brachioradialis muscle. Hemostasis is significantly more difficult when having to compress the muscle to compress the artery, and the risk of hematoma formation is increased. This transition is well up the arm, and the muscle is easily palpated. However, in the unlikely event that multiple access attempts are made that cause spasm, once the muscle is encountered, further attempts at accessing the radial artery when it dives deep to the muscle should be avoided and alternative access sites (ulnar) should be pursued.

Ultrasound Guidance

By far the most important factor of fast and successful cannulation of the radial artery is consistent use of ultrasound for access. Early on in our experience, the senior author felt that ultrasound added time to the procedure. We quickly realized that this was not only incorrect, but that the opposite was true: consistent use of ultrasound dramatically speeds access and lowers complications. This has even been recently shown in a large randomized multicenter controlled trial of over 600 patients, where ultrasound guidance was associated with a significantly lower number of attempts and time to access, as well as improved first-pass success.[9] This reduction in attempts is important in decreasing the likelihood of radial artery vasospasm as well as preventing patient pain, swelling, and hematomas at the access site.[9]

Arterial Puncture and Sheath Placement

Under ultrasound guidance, a 20-gauge needle is advanced into the radial artery (Figure 2.9). If pulsatile, arterial blood is seen exiting the needle, the operator may proceed by advancing a 0.025 inch hydrophilic guide wire through the needle into the artery. This is referred to as a single-wall puncture.[4] Standard technique for femoral access uses single-wall puncture at the level of the femoral artery to avoid a source for hemorrhage. However, the radial artery is a smaller target with a lower risk of hemorrhage. Thus, many operators prefer a double-wall puncture (the original Seldinger technique) for transradial access wherein the needle is passed through both the anterior and posterior wall of the artery.[4] Rather than a standard needle, the double-wall technique is facilitated by use of a needle inside an angiocatheter, both of which often come packaged with the radial sheaths. A small flash of blood will be seen in the hub of the needle as you pass through the artery and the operator should continue to advance the needle after this flash. The operator then withdraws the needle and slowly withdraws the angiocatheter until pulsatile arterial blood flow

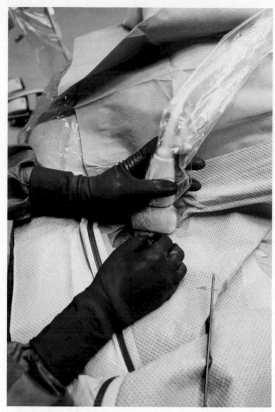

FIGURE 2.9 *Under ultrasound guidance, a 20-gauge needle is advanced into the radial artery with either a single-wall or dual-wall technique.*

is seen. During this maneuver, the tip of the microwire is placed at the hub of the needle in preparation for immediate advancement once pulsatile blood is encountered. The angiocatheter will orient coaxially with the radial artery and the guide wire can be passed through it (Figure 2.10). Bernat et al. found that the double-wall technique was significantly faster and more likely to result in a successful first-pass attempt as compared with the single-wall puncture technique.[10]

Advancement of the guide wire through the needle without visualizing pulsatile blood is not recommended as the tip of the needle is likely extraluminal and can thus lead to discomfort for the patient and arterial vasospasm via manipulation of the adventitia. If there is any concern regarding the position of the wire, ultrasound or fluoroscopy can be performed to evaluate wire position. Under fluoroscopy, if the wire is intraluminal, it will often appear straight with the tip frequently seen in the mid-forearm (Figure 2.11). Once the guide wire is in place, the needle is removed, and the desired introducer sheath can be advanced over the guide wire (Figure 2.12). During this step, careful attention must be paid to ensure that the guide wire is not inadvertently advanced too far forward into the radial artery such that it cannot be retrieved. In order to prevent this, a section of

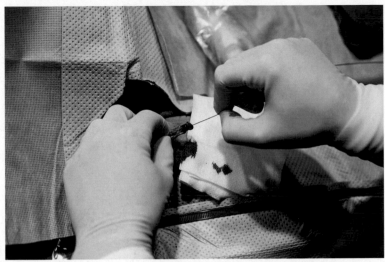

FIGURE 2.10 *With a dual-wall technique, the operator withdraws the needle. Then the angiocatheter is slowly withdrawn until pulsatile arterial blood flow is seen. During this maneuver, the tip of the microwire is placed at the hub of the needle for immediate advancement once pulsatile blood is encountered.*

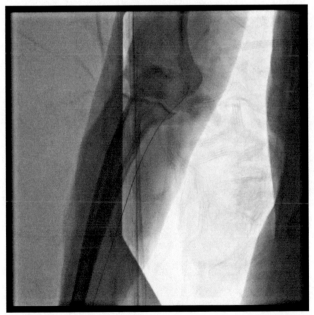

FIGURE 2.11 *Under fluoroscopy, if the wire is intraluminal, it will appear straight with the tip in the mid-forearm.*

guide wire longer than the length of the sheath is typically left outside of the artery so that as the sheath is advanced over the wire, the distal end of the wire can be identified prior to introducing the sheath into the artery. Once the sheath is in place, the guide wire and style are removed and it is secured to the wrist with a tegaderm.

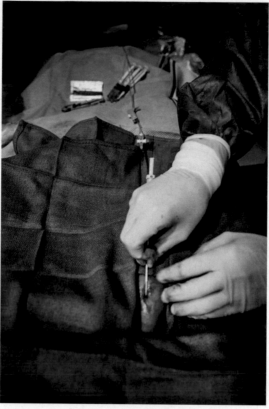

FIGURE 2.12 *Once the guide wire is in place, the needle is removed, and the desired introducer sheath can be advanced over the guide wire.*

Radial Vascular Sheaths

The newer radial slender sheaths have a thinner wall and thus a smaller outer diameter than the femoral conventional sheaths. For example, a 6 French slender sheath has a 6 French inner diameter, yet maintains the same outer diameter as a standard 5 French because the sheath wall measures 0.12 mm rather than the standard 0.20 mm. 5 French slender sheaths are typically used for transradial angiography, and 7 French slender sheaths are usually the largest that most radial arteries can accommodate for interventions with an outer diameter of 2.95 mm and an inner diameter of 2.79 mm. The Terumo slender sheaths (Terumo, Somerset, NJ) are available in 10 or 16 cm lengths, and the Merit radial sheaths are available in 7, 11, or 23 cm lengths (Merit, Salt Lake City, UT). Longer slender sheaths are beneficial in diminishing repetitive friction of catheter movement against the radial artery, which can cause radial artery spasm.

We have significantly increased our use of the longer 23 cm sheaths in our practice. Some operators use them in every case, but we at least check the radial angiogram with

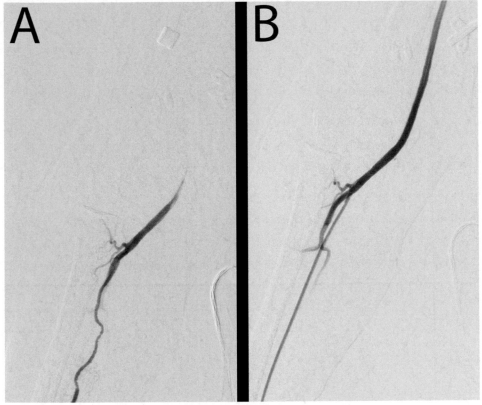

FIGURE 2.13 *After placement of a short transradial sheath, a small radial artery with vasospasm was noted on the radial angiogram (A). The decision was made to place a longer 23 cm sheath which terminates at the brachial bifurcation, obviating the need for navigation of the small spastic artery with the catheters and wires.*

the short sheath to confirm the artery is big enough to accommodate a 5, 6, or 7F guide without spasm. If there is any concern, the short sheath is simply exchanged out for a 23 cm sheath. This length consistently places you in the brachial artery, which completely eliminates the possibility of spasm as the entire length of the radial artery is protected by the hydrophilic sheath. In our experience, the vast majority of patients can accommodate even the 7F 23 cm slender radial sheaths without issue. Figure 2.13 demonstrates a case where the initial radial angiogram revealed a small radial artery (A), prompting us to exchange the short sheath for a longer 23 cm sheath (B), enabling complete coverage of the radial artery and obviating spasm on the diagnostic catheter.

Intraprocedural Medications

After the sheath is in place, the antispasmodic agents (usually 2.5 mg of verapamil and 200 μg of nitroglycerin) are given through the sheath in an effort to prevent radial artery vasospasm (Figure 2.14).[5,11-16] It is important to dilute these medications with blood and to administer them slowly, especially in the awake patient, as they can cause a transient burning sensation in the arm that can lead to significant discomfort when given too quickly. We then administer 65–70 units per kilogram of heparin given intra-arterially or intravenously to protect against postprocedural radial artery occlusion.[17]

Angiography of the Arm

Once good backflow of blood has been identified, an angiogram is performed through the sheath to evaluate for any radial or brachial anatomic abnormalities that may prevent advancement of the catheter into the subclavian artery. While it can be tempting to advance the guide wire and catheter blindly, radial anomalies exist in up to 10% of cases in large series, and every patient should have at least one radial angiogram to

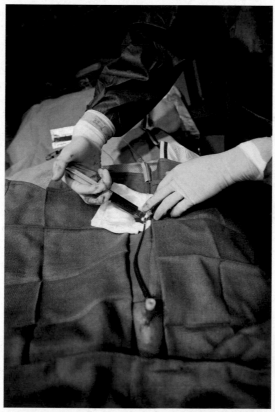

FIGURE 2.14 *After the sheath is in place, the antispasmodic agents (usually 2.5 mg of verapamil and 200 μg of nitroglycerin) are given through the sheath in an effort to prevent radial artery vasospasm. It is important to dilute these medications with blood and to administer them slowly, as they can cause a transient burning sensation in the arm.*

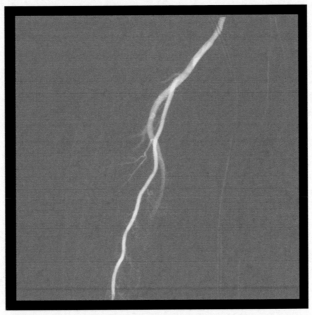

FIGURE 2.15 *Radial road map that should be obtained to elucidate any radial anomalies and facilitate navigation of the guide wire to the subclavian artery.*

confirm their anatomy. Identification and management of radial artery anomalies such has high bifurcation and radial artery loops are further discussed in Chapter 10. The angiogram can also be used as a roadmap for the catheter to avoid lodging the guide wire into smaller arterial branches during access to the subclavian (Figure 2.15).[4] The radial artery angiogram should be performed with only the anteroposterior plane brought head side. Depending on the patient's body habitus, the table may occasionally need to be rotated 5–10 degrees away from the operator in order to properly capture the brachial bifurcation.

RADIAL ARTERY ACCESS FAILURES AND VASOSPASM

Challenges and complications of radial artery access are discussed in Chapter 10. However, in brief, radial artery access failures are usually secondary to errors in technique and/or radial artery spasm from manipulation. Utilizing ultrasound can reduce the number of puncture attempts and thus prevent vasospasm from occurring.[9] In the event that the artery spasms upon attempting to puncture, further attempts can be made more proximal along the radial artery until approximately 2–3 cm cephalad to the radial styloid, where it dives deep to the brachioradialis muscle, making postprocedural hemostasis difficult.[18] If the sheath is able to be placed but significant spasm is seen on the radial angiogram or encountered when advancing the catheter, then additional medications or a longer sheath can considered to bypass the spasm.

REFERENCES

1. Patel A, Naides AI, Patel R, et al. Transradial intervention: basics. *J Vasc Interv Radiol.* 2015;26(5):722.

2. McCarthy DJ, Chen SH, Brunet MC, et al. Distal radial artery access in the anatomical snuffbox for neu-rointerventions: case report. *World Neurosurg.* 2019;122:355–359.

3. Barros G, Bass DI, Osbun JW, et al. Left transradial access for cerebral angiography. *J Neurointerv Surg.* 2020;12(4):427–430. doi:10.1136/neurintsurg-2019-015386.

4. Layton KF, Kallmes DF, Cloft HJ. The radial artery access site for interventional neuroradiology proce-dures. *Am J Neuroradiol.* 2006;27(5):1151–1154.

5. Brunet MC, Chen SH, Sur S, et al. Distal transradial access in the anatomical snuffbox for diagnostic ce-rebral angiography. *J Neurointerv Surg.* 2019;11(7):710–713.

6. Valsecchi O, Vassileva A, Cereda AF, et al. Early clinical experience with right and left distal transradial access in the anatomical snuffbox in 52 consecutive patients. *J Invasive Cardiol.* 2018;30(6):218–223.

7. Al-Azizi KM, Lotfi AS. The distal left radial artery access for coronary angiography and intervention: a new era. *Cardiovasc Revasc Med.* 2018;19(8S):35–40.

8. Soydan E, Akin M. Coronary angiography using the left distal radial approach—an alternative site to conventional radial coronary angiography. *Anatol J Cardiol.* 2018;19(4):243–248.

9. Seto AH, Roberts JS, Abu-Fadel MS, et al. Real-time ultrasound guidance facilitates transradial access: RAUST (Radial Artery access with Ultrasound Trial). *JACC Cardiovasc Interv.* 2015;8(2):283–291.

10. Bernat I, Abdelaal E, Plourde G, et al. Early and late outcomes after primary percutaneous coronary in-tervention by radial or femoral approach in patients presenting in acute ST-elevation myocardial infarc-tion and cardiogenic shock. *Am Heart J.* 2013;165(3):338–343.

11. Brunet MC, Chen SH, Peterson EC. Transradial access for neurointerventions: management of access challenges and complications. *J Neurointerv Surg.* 2020;12:82–86.

12. Chen SH, McCarthy DJ, Sheinberg D, et al. Pipeline embolization device for the treatment of intracra-nial pseudoaneurysms. *World Neurosurg.* 2019;127:e86–e93.

13. Chen SH, Snelling BM, Shah SS, et al. Transradial approach for flow diversion treatment of cerebral aneurysms: a multicenter study. *J Neurointerv Surg.* 2019;11(8):796–800.

14. Chen SH, Snelling BM, Sur S, et al. Transradial versus transfemoral access for anterior circula-tion mechanical thrombectomy: comparison of technical and clinical outcomes. *J Neurointerv Surg.* 2019;11(9):874–878.

15. Snelling BM, Sur S, Shah SS, et al. Transradial approach for complex anterior and posterior circulation interventions: technical nuances and feasibility of using current devices. *Oper Neurosurg (Hagerstown).* 2019;17(3):293–302.

16. Snelling BM, Sur S, Shah SS, et al. Transradial cerebral angiography: techniques and outcomes. *J Neurointerv Surg.* 2018;10(9):874–881.

17. Spaulding C, Lefevre T, Funck F, et al. Left radial approach for coronary angiography: results of a pro-spective study. *Cathet Cardiovasc Diagn.* 1996;39(4):365–370.

18. Blitz A, Osterday RM, Brodman RF. Harvesting the radial artery. *Ann Cardiothorac Surg.* 2013;2(4):533–542.

CHAPTER 3

Distal Transradial "Snuffbox" Approach

MARIE-CHRISTINE BRUNET, STEPHANIE H. CHEN, PASCAL M. JABBOUR, AND ERIC C. PETERSON

ANATOMY OF THE DISTAL RADIAL ARTERY

The radial artery, along with the ulnar artery, is a terminal branch of the brachial artery and usually arises at the intercondylar line of the humerus, a fixed line representing the proximal border of the antecubital fossa. The radial artery runs along the radial aspect of the anterior compartment of the forearm under the brachioradialis, lateral to the flexor carpi radialis tendon. For the distal section of its course, the radial artery lies on the surface of the radius. The radial artery proceeds along the floor of the anatomical snuffbox (AS), passing dorsally around the scaphoid and trapezium. The AS is a depressed space located in the radial part of the wrist and surrounded laterally by the tendons of the abductor pollicis longus and extensor pollicis brevis muscles and medially by the tendon of the extensor pollicis longus muscle. The distal radius, scaphoid, trapezium, and the base of the first metacarpal bone constitute the base of this triangular area. The distal part of the radial artery passes in deep fashion through the AS and continues distally as the deep palmar arch of the hand, which forms anastomosis with the ulnar artery. The notable feature of the distal radial artery segment is its location distal to the origin of the superficial palmar branch of the radial artery, which forms

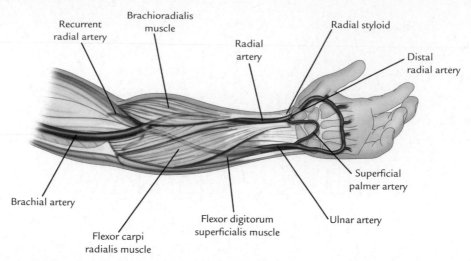

FIGURE 3.1 *Depiction of the vascular supply of the hand demonstrating the palmar arches with contributions from both the radial and ulnar artery. Of note, the distal radial artery segment is distal to the origin of the superficial palmar branch of the radial artery, which forms collaterals with the deep palmar arch.*

collaterals with the deep palmar arch (Figure 3.1). The radial artery provides blood supply to the elbow joint, lateral forearm muscles, radial nerve, carpal bones and joints, thumb, and lateral side of the index finger.

ADVANTAGES OF DISTAL RADIAL ACCESS

1. *Decreases risk of hand ischemia.* The distal transradial approach (dTRA) puncture site is distal to the origin of the superficial palmar branch, which has anastomoses with the ulnar artery to form the superficial palmar arch. This anatomic advantage combined with the low risk of occlusion in the proximal segment results in preservation of blood flow to the fingers and thumb to protect the hand from ischemia.[1–5]

2. *Preservation of the traditional radial access site.* Adopting dTRA as the default access site maintains the proximal radial artery as a back-up option in case of access failure or for future procedures where a larger system might be required, or in the event of an occlusion at the distal site from the initial angiogram. Crossover from dTRA to proximal transradial approach (TRA) should be considered prior to converting to a femoral approach. The two most common reasons for crossover from dTRA to traditional proximal TRA are distal radial artery spasm and small-caliber distal radial artery (generally <1.8 mm diameter).[6]

3. *More ergonomic for patient.* dTRA also confers ergonomic advantages compared to TRA because there is no need for hand supination. The arm can rest

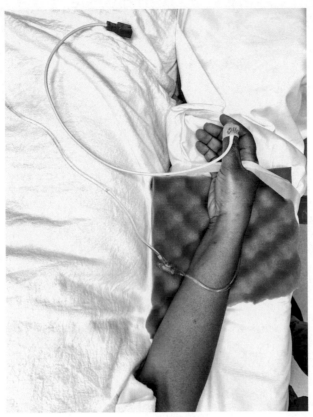

FIGURE 3.2 *Distal transradial access positioning of the hand with the arm resting in neutral position.*

in a neutral position, which is more comfortable for the patient (Figure 3.2). This is particularly beneficial in elderly patients with orthopedic limitations. Koutouzis et al. found that patient satisfaction trended higher in the dTRA than TRA groups, although the difference was not significant.[7] Moreover, since full supination can force the hand laterally, the neutral position of dTRA eases the adduction of the arm against the patient's hip, creating a more favorable set-up for catheter and wire placement and facilitating forearm navigation under fluoroscopy with minimal or no lateral angulation of the table (Figure 3.3).

4. *Facilitates left-sided catheterization.* When using left dTRA, the operator stands at the right side of the patient and the natural hand position of dTRA also allows for simple left-sided dTRA with the hand draped across the body with no need to lean over the patient's abdomen to reach the left arm (Figure 3.4). This option may be particularly useful in cases where the left vertebral artery is dominant or in cases of a challenging vertebral artery origin angle from transfemoral approach (TFA) or right TRA.[6]

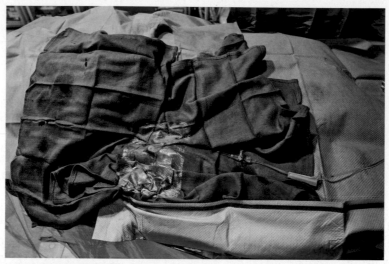

FIGURE 3.3 *The patient is draped with the arm against the patient's hip, and all catheters and wires rest on padding caudal to the hand.*

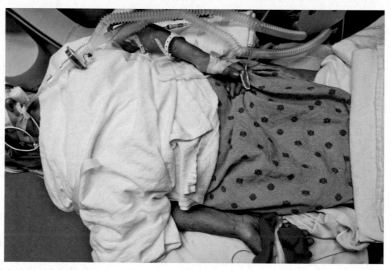

FIGURE 3.4 *For left distal transradial access, the operator stands on the right side of the patient, and the hand is draped across the body and allowed to rest in its natural position.*

5. *Faster hemostasis with distal radial access.* The location of the carpal bones relative to the access site facilitates hemostasis with light compression, thereby providing an advantage over proximal radial access at the wrist. The radius bone is at an oblique angle relative to the radial artery versus the horizontal plane of the carpal bones, making TRA hemostasis less effective and more prone to bleeding. As a result, hemostatic wrist bands require twice the amount of air and longer duration of compression to achieve homeostasis after TRA compared with dTRA. Koutouzis et al. found a significantly shorter postprocedural duration of hemostasis.[7]

STEP-BY-STEP TECHNIQUE FOR DISTAL TRANSRADIAL ACCESS

Similar to standard radial access, topical 2.5% lidocaine/prilocaine cream is applied to the distal radial artery area in the wrist and forearm and covered with an adhesive dressing for 15–30 minutes prior to the start of the procedure. The patient is positioned with the hand tightly against the hip, and bolsters are added both inferior and caudal to the hand to allow a consistent platform on which to rest the catheters and wires. Notably, in contrast to traditional TRA, for dTRA the hand is allowed to lie in its natural position with the palm facing the hip. A slight ulnar abduction is achieved by curling the thumb into the other four fingers, thus forcing the fossa radialis upward.

The periarterial tissue is infiltrated with 2 cc of lidocaine. While use of ultrasound is strongly recommended for TRA after the Radial Artery Access with Ultrasound Trial (RAUST) showed it lowers time to access and complications,[8] ultrasound is even more necessary for fast and consistent access in dTRA. A 20-gauge needle is angled 45–50 degrees medially in the direction of the radial artery and the anterior wall of the artery is punctured. Upon brisk blood return, a 0.025 hydrophilic guide wire is threaded into the radial artery, and a 5F Glidesheath Slender 10 cm (Terumo, Somerset, NJ) is placed into the radial artery. Antispasmolytic agents (verapamil 2.5 mg and nitroglycerine 200 µg) are infused in the sheath, and 4000 units of heparin are administered intravenously. Similar to TFA, access is obtained with only the anteroposterior plane in position. As the arm is closer to the body than in standard TRA, often rotation of the table is not necessary to visualize the right forearm under anteroposterior monoplane. The remainder of the case proceeds in an identical fashion to standard TRA.

Closure is performed with the DistalSync closure band (Merit, Salt Lake City, UT) (Figure 3.5). After inflation, release of small amounts of air from the device is done until a small amount of bleeding occurs, after which we inject another 1 cc of air. By using the minimum amount of compression needed for hemostasis, we maximize the chances of preserved radial artery patency.[6] As with the proximal TRA site, with careful attention to patent hemostasis technique, the dTRA site can be reaccessed repeatedly.

LEARNING CURVE

Mastering dTRA is associated with an appreciable learning curve due to the more angulated trajectory of the distal radial artery as compared to the straight trajectory of the proximal radial artery. In a recent study, Brunet et al. reported their initial experience with dTRA for cerebral angiography and observed an initial inability to insert the wire despite brisk blood flow from the cannula. However, they found that aiming the needle 45–50

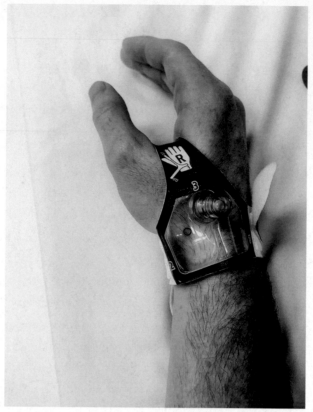

FIGURE 3.5 *Patent hemostasis is performed using an inflatable DistalSync closure band (Merit, Salt Lake City, UT).*

degrees medially toward the course of the distal radial artery (which can be traced with ultrasound) corrected that problem. They reported a total failure rate of 8.2%. Notably, in the first and second quarters, they experienced a 14.3% conversion to traditional TRA or TFA. However, in the third quarter, the failure rate decreased to 4.7% and to 0% in the last (fourth) quarter.[6] That steeper learning curve may make some interventionalists reluctant to incorporate this new technique; however, patient preference and preservation of the radial artery are accelerating the transition from "radial first" to "distal radial first."

REFERENCES

1. Orazio V, Alberto FC, Alfonso E, et al. Early clinical experience with right and left distal transradial access in the anatomical snuffbox in 52 consecutive patients. *J Invasive Cardiol.* 2018;30:218–223.
2. Babunashvili A. TCT-810 Novel distal transradial approach for coronary and peripheral interventions. *J Am Coll Cardiol.* 2018;72(13):B323.
3. Al-Azizi KM, Grewal V, Gobeil K, et al. The left distal trans-radial artery access for coronary angiography and intervention: a US experience. *Cardiovasc Revasc Med.* 2019;20(9):786–789. doi:10.1016/j.carrev.2018.10.023.

4. Soydan E. Coronary angiography using the left distal radial approach—an alternative site to conventional radial coronary angiography. *Anatol J Cardiol.* 2018;19(4):243–248.

5. Mizuguchi Y, Izumikawa T, Hashimoto S, et al. Efficacy and safety of the distal transradial approach in coronary angiography and percutaneous coronary intervention: a Japanese multicenter experience. *Cardiovasc Interv and Ther.* 2020;35:162–167. https://doi.org/10.1007/s12928-019-00590-0

6. Brunet MC, Chen SH, Sur S, et al. Distal transradial access in the anatomical snuffbox for diagnostic cerebral angiography. *J Neurointerv Surg.* 2019;11:710–713.

7. Koutouzis M, Kontopodis E, Tassopoulos A, et al. Distal versus traditional radial approach for coronary angiography. *Cardiovasc Revasc Med.* 2019;20(8):678–680. doi:10.1016/j.carrev.2018.09.018

8. Seto AH, Roberts JS, Abu-Fadel MS, et al. Real-time ultrasound guidance facilitates transradial access: RAUST (Radial Artery access with Ultrasound Trial). *JACC Cardiovasc Interv.* 2015;8(2):283–291. doi:10.1016/j.jcin.2014.05.036

CHAPTER 4

Diagnostic Angiography

JONATHON LEBOVITZ, CHRISTOPHER STOREY, ERIC C. PETERSON, AND PASCAL M. JABBOUR

TRANSRADIAL ANGIOGRAPHY CAN PROVIDE THE SAME HIGH-QUALITY pictures that can be achieved via a transfemoral approach using the existing catheters and techniques.[1–3] The goal is to achieve the same results as the transfemoral approach with the improved safety and comfort profile that transradial access provides. The two most popular ways are traditional radial access versus distal transradial or snuffbox access. Positioning is shown in the following Figures 4.1 to 4.7.

When imaging the posterior fossa is of interest, we prefer to obtain images by first catheterizing the right vertebral artery. Not only is it the first artery of interest encountered, but it also allows you to see exactly what quality left vertebral injection is needed. If you inject the right vertebral artery on the way out and then need to go back for better left vertebral artery pictures, then the Simmons catheter will have to be shaped again. We want to decrease the number of times that the Simmons catheter has to be shaped.

After navigating your catheter to the arch, the next step is to select the vessels of interest. There are times when the glide wire will select the right common carotid artery without going into the aortic arch first (Figure 4.E). When this happens, we recommend that you continue to push your wire close to the carotid bifurcation and allow the diagnostic catheter to track into the common carotid artery. This maneuver usually will leave the catheter in a stable position for you to go on to select the internal and/or external

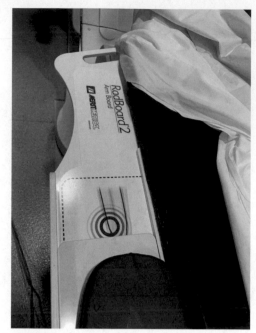

FIGURE 4.1 *Radial board.*

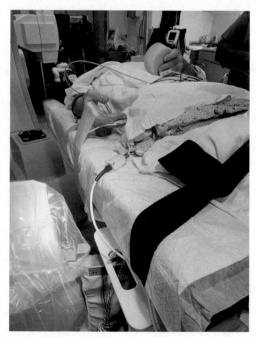

FIGURE 4.2 *Hand position after building up the platform.*

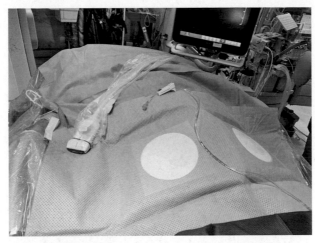

FIGURE 4.4 *Draping and ultrasound.*

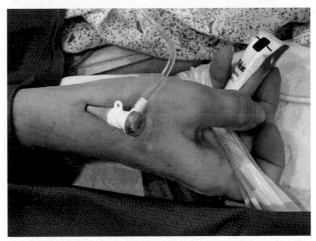

FIGURE 4.3 *Neutral anatomical position with the thumb pointing upward in the case of distal transradial, anatomical snuffbox.*

carotid artery under road map guidance. After completing the imaging of the right side, we recommend that you pull the catheter back into the common carotid artery and subsequently push the catheter back into the arch to maintain its shape (Figure 4.A). With tortuosity it may not push into the arch and may tract the carotid, and you must keep a careful eye on this for fear of causing a dissection. If this is noted, pull back and twist while you are pushing.

For the majority of cases, the Simmons catheter will needed to be shaped either in the ascending or descending aorta (Figure 4.B). When you are unable to shape the Simmons catheter in the usual way, there are a few tricks to get the catheter into position. The first technique utilizes pushing the glide wire and letting it bounce on the aortic valve. This

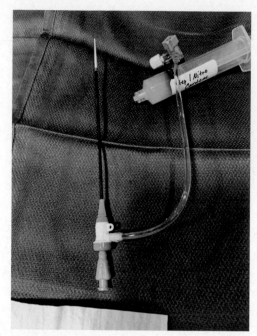

FIGURE 4.5 *Merit Prelude radial sheath.*

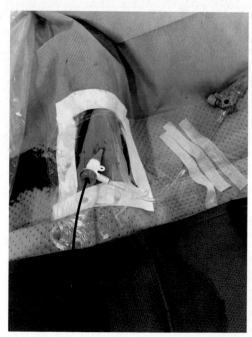

FIGURE 4.6 *Simmons 2 Penumbra inserted in the radial sheath.*

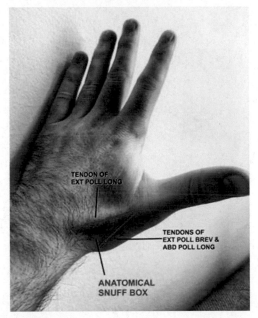

FIGURE 4.7 *The anatomical snuffbox.*

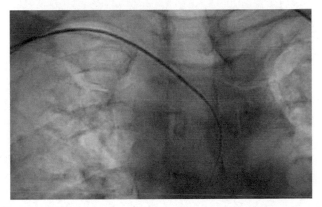

FIGURE 4.A *Forming the Simmons 2 catheter.*

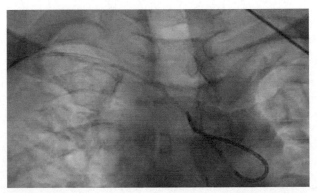

FIGURE 4.B *Simmons 2 formed.*

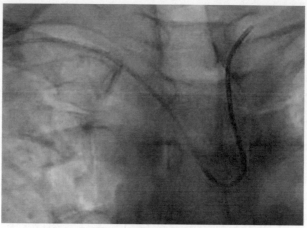

FIGURE 4.C *Selecting the left common carotid artery.*

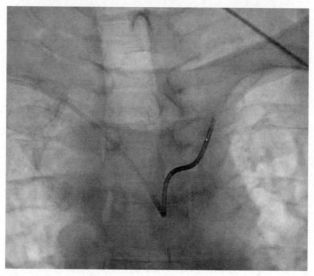

FIGURE 4.D *Selecting the left vertebral artery.*

should allow you to push the catheter over the wire into the correct shape. Another option is to reformat the catheter in the descending aorta.

It tends to work best if you work from left to right once you enter the arch. If you have
just injected the right vertebral artery, the head will be at the correct level for another
posterior fossa run once the left vertebral artery is selected. We always leave a cuff on the
left arm or have a Simmons 3 catheter ready to aid in performing a subclavian injection or
catheterizing the left vertebral artery (Figure 4.D).

Then we proceed to the left carotid artery followed by the right carotid artery (Figure
4.C). These injections should be performed based on necessity and anatomy as you would
perform from a femoral approach. As with a femoral approach, sometimes tortuosity

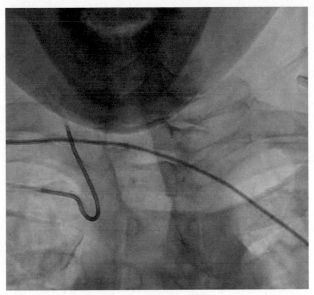

FIGURE 4.E *Selecting the right common carotid artery.*

does not allow you to climb for internal or external selective injections. If images are inadequate, a femoral approach in some cases provides easier selectivity for the left carotid, but with experience and as technology improves, these cases should become rare. There are also times when you have a difficult type 3 arch where a standard Berenstein catheter may work better to get the left carotid artery. When this is the case, if you have a good road map, you can exchange your Simmons catheter over a wire for a Berenstein or angled catheter. These angled catheters can be advanced over the glide wire and should offer enough support to allow the catheter to select the internal and/or external artery.

Any radial case runs the risk of spasm that can cause significant resistance of catheter movement. There are several options. The first step should be injection of additional doses of calcium channel blockers to vasodilate the artery. If the catheter can be removed, it can be exchanged with a long radial sheath so that the hydrophilic coating extends to the brachial artery. Proceeding with the angiogram with increasing resistance increases the risk of worsening spasm and kinking the catheter, which could lead to the worst-case scenario of a retained catheter. If the catheter becomes immobile, it is imperative that it be placed on flush while it is attempted to be removed. If calcium channel blockers do not improve catheter movement, a cuff can be inflated to tourniquet level pressure and clamped for 10 minutes. This tissue ischemia will lead to localized vasodilation and aid in catheter release. The catheter can usually be removed with slow, steady pressure with these maneuvers. Also, it is important to fluoroscopy the entire length of the catheter for kinks that may have developed proximally due to distal spasm that can accordion the thin radial sheath.

Following these steps can allow you to become as efficient with radial as with any femoral case with a type 3 arch. To become efficient, one has to commit to radial access as there is a learning curve.[4-7] With the tips provided in this chapter we hope that we can significantly shorten your learning curve.

REFERENCES

1. Matsumoto Y, Hongo K, Toriyama T, Nagashima H, Kobayashi S. Transradial approach for diagnostic selective cerebral angiography: results of a consecutive series of 166 cases. *AJNR Am J Neuroradiol.* 2001;22(4):704–708.
2. Sgueglia GA, Di Giorgio A, Gaspardone A, Babunashvili A. Anatomic basis and physiological rationale of distal radial artery access for percutaneous coronary and endovascular procedures. *JACC: Cardiov Interv.* 2018;11(20):2113–2119.
3. Yoo B-S, Yoon J, Ko J-Y, et al. Anatomical consideration of the radial artery for transradial coronary procedures: arterial diameter, branching anomaly and vessel tortuosity. *Int J Cardiol.* 2005;101(3):421–427.
4. Levy EI, Boulos AS, Fessler RD, et al. Transradial cerebral angiography: an alternative route. *Neurosurgery.* 2002;51(2):335–340;discussion 340–332.
5. Matsumoto Y, Hokama M, Nagashima H, et al. Transradial approach for selective cerebral angiography: technical note. *Neurol Res.* 2000;22(6):605–608.
6. Jo KW, Park SM, Kim SD, Kim SR, Baik MW, Kim YW. Is transradial cerebral angiography feasible and safe? A single center's experience. *J Korean Neurosurg Soc.* 2010;47(5):332–337.
7. Pancholy SB, Sanghvi KA, Patel TM. Radial artery access technique evaluation trial: randomized comparison of Seldinger versus modified Seldinger technique for arterial access for transradial catheterization. *Catheter Cardiovasc Interv.* 2012;80(2):288–291.

CHAPTER 5

Transradial Interventional Procedures

BRIAN SNELLING, STEPHANIE H. CHEN,
PASCAL M. JABBOUR, AND ERIC C. PETERSON

INTRODUCTION

The utilization of the transradial approach (TRA) for neurovascular interventional procedures confers many benefits for the operator, patient, and staff.[1-10] The decrease in major access-site complications is particularly beneficial in interventional procedures compared to cerebral angiography, due to the use of larger-bore sheaths and catheters, anticoagulation, and frequent use of dual antiplatelet therapy. Furthermore, the patient preference benefits of TRA are not specific to cerebral angiography, as patients are able to sit and ambulate more quickly following extubation with TRA compared to the transfemoral approach (TFA). This chapter describes the clinical and technical considerations necessary for successful completion of neurovascular interventions from TRA.

PATIENT SELECTION

Clinical Characteristics That Favor the Transradial Approach

Clinical characteristics that favor TRA, beyond the benefits outlined in the first chapter of this book, can broadly be thought of as any factors that may increase the likelihood of access-site complications if TFA were to be used. This includes patients currently taking oral anticoagulant or antiplatelet medications (including those administered during the procedure), obese patients, patients with known peripheral arterial disease of the lower extremities, those with aorto-iliac occlusive disease, patients with prior vascular surgery or intervention to the descending aorta or iliac or femoral arteries, or patients with prior surgery in the inguinal area.[1,2,11–15] Furthermore, TRA is favored in patients where early ambulation is important post procedure, including the elderly, patients with low back pain, and patients with hereditary or acquired thombophilias at risk for deep vein thrombosis. Finally, TRA is favored in pregnant patients because it may lessen radiation exposure to the gravid uterus during the procedure, as the abdomen can be covered with a lead drape.[16]

Clinical Characteristics That Do Not Favor the Transradial Approach

TRA should be avoided in patients with Raynaud's phenomenon, reflex sympathetic dystrophy of the upper extremity ipsilateral to site of access, presence of an ipsilateral upper-extremity arteriovenous dialysis fistula, or prior extremity trauma.

Anatomical Characteristics That Favor the Transradial Approach

Interventions of the posterior circulation, where the target artery for guide catheter placement is the vertebral artery or subclavian artery (such as vertebral artery origin stenting), are ideal for access from the radial artery *ipsilateral to target artery* (e.g., left radial artery access if the intended target artery is the left vertebral artery).[17,18] Thus, the guide catheter can be placed without entering the aortic arch. This avoids iatrogenic emboli from the aortic arch (an inherent risk of catheter manipulation within the arch regardless of access site). Furthermore, it also confers additional stability as the catheter is maintained within smaller diameter vessels (radial, brachial, and subclavian arteries) en route to the target artery as opposed to the capacious aorta. This serves as an anatomical "sheath," which provides further guide catheter stability.

Similarly, this principle can be extended to the anterior circulation as well. Interventions of the right carotid arteries (common carotid artery [CCA], internal carotid artery [ICA], or external carotid artery [ECA]) similarly avoid placement of the guide catheter into the aortic arch (though the Simmons 2 diagnostic and guide catheters occasionally have to be introduced into the aortic arch to form the Simmons 2 shape and select the right CCA if the right CCA cannot be selected directly from the brachiocephalic trunk). Additionally, in the setting of a bovine aortic arch, this principle further applies to the target artery of the left carotid arteries. The bovine aortic arch variant if often able to be selected directly from the brachiocephalic trunk—without Simmons 2 diagnostic catheter formation—and confers a favorable angle when compared to TFA (Figure 5.1).

CHOICE OF GUIDE CATHETER AND TRANSRADIAL SHEATH

The choice of guide catheter to be used depends upon several factors: the patient's radial artery diameter, type of neurovascular intervention to be performed, target artery for intervention, aortic arch and target vessel anatomy, and support requirements for the case.

Radial Artery Diameter

Radial artery diameter can limit the placement of larger guide catheters and sheaths. The radial diameter is much smaller in diameter compared to the femoral artery, and as such, the size of the radial artery must be taken into account when deciding choice of guide catheter. This is due to the fact that, while universally clinically asymptomatic, radial artery occlusion (RAO) rates significantly increase when the diameter of the sheath (or guide catheter if placed sheathlessly) exceeds the diameter of the radial artery.[19-22] In addition, entrapment of the catheter can occur within the radial artery due to severe radial artery spasm from an oversized catheter.

Although hand ischemia from RAO is an extremely rare phenomenon, preservation of radial artery patency is important in order to be able to utilize the radial artery as an access point for future angiography and interventions.[23,24] This principle, while certainly important, must also be weighed in the balance of being able to quickly and successfully complete a life-saving, emergency neurovascular procedure (such as mechanical thrombectomy) with the appropriate catheters and devices via TRA. Thus, if use of a 0.088 inch ID catheter is beneficial in increasing the efficiency and first-pass success of mechanical thrombectomy via TRA, the increased asymptomatic RAO rate is likely a worthwhile trade-off compared to a decreased likelihood of procedural success if a smaller catheter or alternative access site were to be used (Figures 5.2 and 5.3).

Target Artery and Aortic Arch Anatomy

Prior knowledge of the anatomy of the target artery for intervention and aortic arch can provide important information when deciding which catheter system to use. The ability to place the guide catheter into the target artery without traversing into the aortic arch

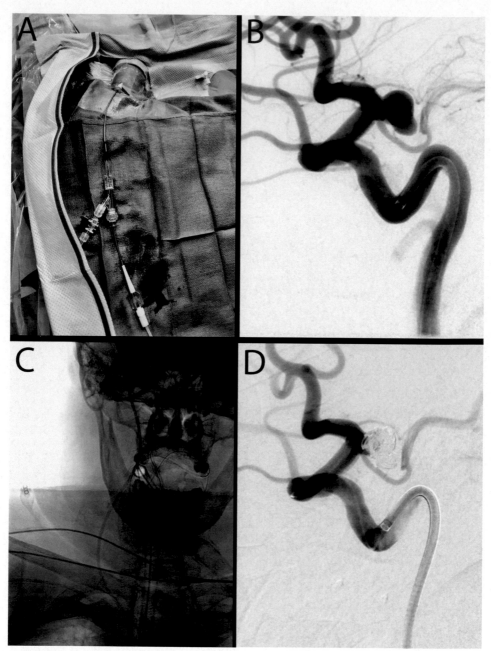

FIGURE 5.1 *(A) A transradial approach with a 6 French slender vascular sheath and 6 French guide catheter was used to perform coil embolization of an (B) irregular posterior communicating artery aneurysm measuring 10 × 8 mm pointing inferiorly and posteriorly. (C) A single shot X-ray of a 6 French guide catheter placed in the right internal carotid artery from a right transradial approach. (D) Successful coiling of right posterior communicating artery aneurysm with Excelsior SL-10 microcatheter (Stryker, Fremont, CA) through the 6 French Benchmark guide catheter (Penumbra, Alameda, CA).*

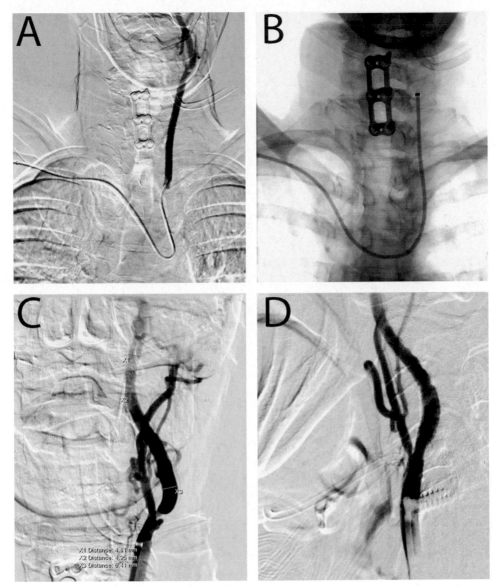

FIGURE 5.2 *Right transradial approach for symptomatic left internal carotid artery (ICA) stenting. (A) Selection of the left common carotid artery with 5 French 130 cm Simmons 2 catheter telescoped through 0.088 inch guide catheter. (B) The 0.088 inch guide catheter is placed into the radial artery sheathless and advanced over the diagnostic catheter into the left common carotid artery. (C) Angiogram demonstrating severe left ICA stenosis at the origin. (D) Successful stenting with 7 × 30 mm Precise stent (Cordis, Santa Clara, CA) of left ICA stenosis.*

provides excellent catheter stability, often better than what can be achieved from a TFA approach. This can be routinely achieved in either vertebral artery (from an ipsilateral TRA approach) or the right carotid arteries (CCA, ICA, or ECA). A bovine aortic arch variant with the left carotid arteries (CCA, ICA, or ECA) as the target vessel provides

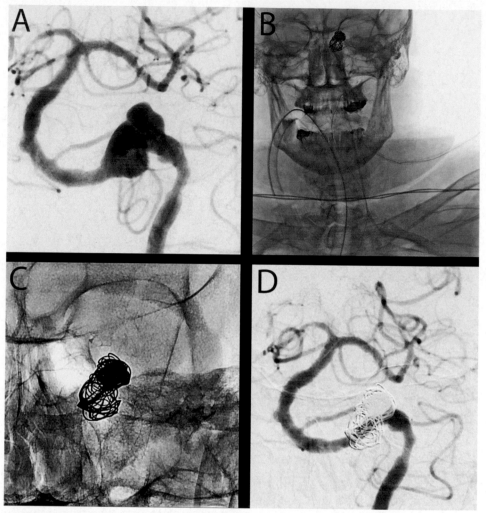

FIGURE 5.3 *Left distal transradial approach for (A) left dominant vertebral dissecting aneurysm. (B) A 0.088 inch guide catheter was placed sheathless in the left distal radial artery and navigated into the left vertebral artery. (C) Flow-diverting stent and coil embolization were performed with a Phenom 0.027 inch microcatheter (Medtronic, Minneapolis, MN) telescoped through a Stryker DAC 0.044 inch catheter (Stryker, Fremont, CA) for flow-diverting stent deployment and an adjacent Headway 0.017 inch microcatheter for coiling (Microvention, Aliso Viejo, CA). (D) Follow-up angiogram 6 months after stent coiling demonstrating obliteration of dissecting aneurysm.*

excellent support for guide catheters, again by utilizing an arterial path that avoids the capacious aortic arch.

If prior angiography or noninvasive imaging reveals the presence of tortuous aortic arch anatomy or dolichoectasia of the target arteries, consideration should be made of placement of a guide catheter larger than the standard 6F size, which will offer more support from a proximal position if it cannot be tracked successfully into the distal target artery.

Case Selection

As a general principle, one cannot dabble in TRA. The willingness to commit a significant majority of one's practice to TRA is required to develop the mastery and proficiency that allow for seamless, efficient use of the technique. Occasional employment of TRA will inevitably result in its use only as a bailout strategy when TFA has failed in emergency cases, which will invariably only result in frustration and abandonment of the technique. Thus, it is also recommended to start with elective cases as opposed to emergencies. At a minimum, the transition should begin with attempting radial first in all posterior circulation interventions and minimal support anterior circulation or ECA interventions (embolization procedures, aneurysm coiling, and assisted coiling procedures). Case selection should then expand to elective interventions requiring more support (carotid and intracranial angioplasty and stenting, flow diversion), with mechanical thrombectomy conquered last. Interventions for large-vessel occlusion require the need for large-bore devices and speed. While the case itself is not technically difficult, the only difficulty of radial for mechanical thrombectomy is building the requisite speed so revascularization times are comparable between TRA and TFA.[4] This can be further stratified into selecting stroke cases that will have faster puncture to revascularization times earlier in one's transition, such as posterior circulation cases, those with type II/III arches, and left-side strokes with bovine arches.

Intervention-Specific Considerations

The entire spectrum of transarterial neurovascular procedures can be performed adequately via TRA.[4,6,25–27] The majority of neurovascular interventions require minimal support and can be completed with a 6F guide catheter. This includes most aneurysm repairs (coiling, balloon-assisted coiling, stent-assisted coiling), embolizations (arteriovenous malformation, tumor, subdural hematoma, epistaxis), and other miscellaneous single-microcatheter procedures.

Interventions that require more support include intracranial angioplasty stenting, intrasaccular flow diversion, and intracranial stenting. Perhaps the greatest support requirements, however, are required for placement of flow-diverting stents. In these cases, consideration must also be made for the need of an intermediate catheter, often needed for intracranial support. If utilizing a 6F guide catheter, the tolerance between the 0.071 inch ID of the guide catheter, such as Benchmark or Envoy DA, and an 0.058 inch ID intermediate catheter (Navien, Medtronic, Irvine, CA) is occasionally too small to allow for placement. In these cases, a smaller intermediate catheter such as a 5F Sofia (Microvention, Aliso Viejo, CA) or 0.044 inch Phenom (Medtronic, Irvine, CA) may be utilized. However, when increased intracranial support is thought to be required based on preoperative cerebral angiography, it is recommended to utilize a larger guide catheter, such as a 7F or 8F guide catheter, which can be placed without a vascular sheath into the radial artery.[25]

A special consideration should be made for carotid angioplasty and stenting. These procedures not only require increased support but also require a more unstable position of the guide catheter within the CCA rather than distal placement of the guide in the cervical ICA. Carotid stenting via 6F guide catheters has been reported and is feasible; however, the choice of carotid stent is currently limited to the Precise (Cordis, Santa Clara, CA) stent for a 6F guide catheter. Thus, a low threshold should exist in the setting of tortuous aortic arch and CCA anatomy for utilization of a larger guide catheter, such as 7F or 8F, for these procedures.

Balloon test occlusion (BTO) can be performed with TRA for one or both arterial access sites. If utilizing one TRA and one TFA access site, we recommend placing the smaller sheath and conducting cerebral angiography from the TFA site to mitigate the risk of access-site complications. Utilization of both TRA access sites has been done, conducting cerebral angiography from a left TRA or dTRA site.[28]

Choosing from Currently Available Catheters

It is worthwhile to mention that currently no guide catheter designed for neurovascular access from TRA exists on the market in the United States or abroad. Therefore, all reported neurovascular interventions completed via TRA have utilized guide catheters designed for TFA. As a general principle, these catheters are more similar than unique with respect to their trackability and support characteristics from a TRA approach.

6F catheter options include Benchmark (Penumbra, Alameda, CA), Envoy DA (Cerenovus, J&J, New Brunswick, NJ), and Fubuki (Asahi, Aichi, Japan). In cases where minimal support is required, such as simple posterior circulation interventions, use of 6F Sofia (Microvention, Aliso Viejo, CA) has also been reported.

7F options are more limited due to lack of specific intracranial support or aspiration catheters designed for use with a 7F guide catheter, but options include the Fubuki and Envoy catheters. Of note, 7F slender radial sheaths—GlideSheath Slender (Terumo, Somerset, NJ) and Prelude Ideal (Merit Medical, Salt Lake City, UT)—are available and should be used with these catheters.

8F options require sheathless placement, wherein a 7Fr vascular sheath is exchanged over a wire for the guide catheter. However, this catheter size (0.088 inch ID) supports the full spectrum of intracranial catheters and devices, including large-bore aspiration catheters and coil-assisted flow diversion (utilizing an 0.044 inch ID intracranial support catheter). There are several options, including the Infinity LS (Stryker Neurovascular, Fremont, CA), Ballast (Balt, Irvine, CA), Fubuki (Asahi, Aichi, Japan), NeuronMax (Penumbra, Alameda, CA), or Shuttle sheath (Cook Medical, Bloomington, IN). In our experience, the 0.88 inch Infinity LS offers unique advantages in the sheathless approach, predominantly because it has a longer stylet with less mismatch between the inner diameter of the catheter and the outer diameter of the stylet as compared to other catheters. Significant mismatch can lead to difficulty in transition through the skin as well as a sharp leading edge of the catheter that can injure endothelium.

GUIDE CATHETER PLACEMENT

Catheter Set-up

It is recommended to utilize a biaxial or "telescoped" catheter and wire construct, as opposed to a guide catheter exchange, when performing neurovascular procedures via TRA. Guide catheter exchanges increase catheter manipulation within the radial artery compared to a "telescoped" approach. This increases the risk of radial artery spasm. Furthermore, guide catheter advancement during an exchange poses the risk of intimal injury and dissection due to "step-off" between the guide catheter and wire. This is a risk of not only the target artery, but the radial, brachial, and subclavian arteries as well.

The biaxial setup requires the use of a longer diagnostic Simmons 2 catheter, usually 125 cm or longer, to ensure sufficient length beyond the end of the guide catheter to allow the Simmons 2 catheter to be formed in the aortic arch. If the vertebral artery is the target artery, a Berenstein or vertebral shaped diagnostic catheter, again with a longer length, may also be used and may assist with vertebral catheterization.

Placement of Sheathless Guide Catheter

As previously mentioned, placement of a guide catheter that would require an 8 French sheath—typically those with an inner diameter of 0.088–0.091 inches—requires placement without a sheath ("sheathless") given the size constraints of the radial artery. This process begins with the placement of a 7F slender arterial sheath, either in the standard location proximal to the wrist crease or in the anatomical snuffbox if diameter permits. These access techniques are discussed in detail in Chapters 2 and 3. The 7F slender arterial sheath is then used to perform a radial arteriogram as well as administer a spasmolytic cocktail. The 7F slender sheath is preferred because its tapered hydrophilic coating dilates the arteriotomy to a similar outer diameter as the guide catheter, mitigating the need for a "skin nick" with a scalpel. Under road map guidance of the radial and proximal brachial arteries, a 0.035 inch guide wire is placed into the brachial artery through the sheath. The sheath is removed and the guide catheter—prepared on the back table with its introducer—is advanced into the brachial artery under road map guidance. Care is taken not to advance the tip of the introducer, occasionally poorly visualized, beyond the wire. The introducer is removed, and the diagnostic catheter and guide wire are inserted.

Guide Catheter Navigation to Target Artery

For catheterization of the carotid arteries, a 125 cm Simmons 2 diagnostic catheter should be formed in the aortic arch and used to select the target vessel, as previously described in the angiography chapter. The guide catheter can remain in the brachio-cephalic trunk during diagnostic catheter formation and vessel selection. The CCA is selected with the diagnostic catheter. Under road map guidance, the hydrophilic wire is advanced into the target artery (or the ECA if the CCA is the vessel of choice). The diagnostic catheter is advanced into the target artery over the wire, followed by the guide catheter. Care must be taken to ensure the catheter system is fully apposed to the angle of the aortic arch and target artery ostia to prevent catheter herniation into the aortic arch.

For catheterization of the vertebral artery, ipsilateral TRA should be used. The guide catheter, diagnostic catheter, and hydrophilic wire are advanced to the ipsilateral subclavian artery, and the target vertebral artery is selected with a Berenstein diagnostic catheter under negative road map. The diagnostic catheter is then advanced over the wire, followed by the guide catheter.

TECHNICAL NUANCES

The unique angle to the supra-aortic arterial vasculature combined with the modern neurovascular intervention technical demands of simultaneous trackability and support creates challenges for current transfemoral guide catheters, as there is no available guide catheter currently to access the cerebrovasculature from TRA.

Difficult Guide Catheter Advancement to the Anterior Circulation

Often, there can be difficulty advancing the guide catheter into the CCA over the diagnostic catheter and wire, resulting in herniation of the construct into the aortic arch. Care should be taken to ensure that the guide wire is placed, under road map guidance, as high as safely possible into the ICA (if the ICA is the intended target artery) or ECA (if the CCA or ECA is the target artery). Additionally, care should be taken to ensure that the diagnostic catheter is fully apposed to the wall of the aortic arch to prevent herniation.

If herniation is still noted after these maneuvers, use of a long, stiff glide wire (Terumo IS, Somerset, NJ) or hybrid stiff wire (Terumo Advantage, Terumo IS, Somerset, NJ) will often provide enough support to be able to advance the catheter. Finally, an inspiratory hold or Valsalva maneuver can occasionally straighten tortuous or kinked cervical carotid arteries to allow for guide catheter advancement. Beyond these maneuvers, a combination of guide catheter and diagnostic catheter advancement can be attempted incrementally, though this is often without success.

Difficult Guide Catheter Advancement to the Posterior Circulation

Difficulty in advancement of the guide catheter into the vertebral artery often results from either a proximal origin or a tortuous origin to the vertebral artery—or rarely both. Acute angulation of the vertebral artery origin can make selection with both the guide wire and diagnostic catheter difficult and may not provide sufficient support to advance a guide catheter into its desired location.

In these situations, a microcatheter and microwire in conjunction with an intermediate catheter can be utilized to overcome any difficulty. Under road map or masked guidance, the microcatheter and microwire are advanced in the distal V2 or V3 segment of the vertebral artery. This often provides sufficient support to advance a coaxially placed intermediate catheter. Once the intermediate catheter is in place, the guide catheter can be advanced with minimal risk of intimal injury due to lack of "step-off."

Know When to Cross Over to Femoral Access

Further descriptions of how to overcome transradial-specific challenges are addressed in Chapter 10. However, an important nuance of completing neurovascular interventions from a TRA is understanding that given the current utilization of catheters designed for TFA, a certain subset of cases will not be able to be completed. Crossover rates for interventions range from 5% to 10% depending on the type of case.[4,6,25–28] Preventing crossovers centers on appropriate case selection and sufficient experience. Early recognition of the inability to place the guide catheter to an appropriate position that would allow for equivalent support when compared to TFA is paramount, and it should result in crossover to TFA, especially in time-sensitive or emergency procedures. Crossover rates will reduce with operator experience and future availability of radial-specific neurovascular guide catheters but should be recognized early in order to complete the procedure safely and efficiently.

REFERENCES

1. Alnasser SM, Bagai A, Jolly SS, et al. Transradial approach for coronary angiography and intervention in the elderly: a meta-analysis of 777,841 patients. *Int J Cardiol.* 2017;228:45–51.

2. Cantor WJ, Mehta SR, Yuan F, et al. Radial versus femoral access for elderly patients with acute coronary syndrome undergoing coronary angiography and intervention: insights from the RIVAL trial. *Am Heart J.* 2015;170(5):880–886.

3. Chase AJ, Fretz EB, Warburton WP, et al. Association of the arterial access site at angioplasty with transfusion and mortality: the M.O.R.T.A.L study (Mortality benefit Of Reduced Transfusion after percutaneous coronary intervention via the Arm or Leg). *Heart.* 2008;94(8):1019–1025.

4. Chen SH, Snelling BM, Sur S, et al. Transradial versus transfemoral access for anterior circulation mechanical thrombectomy: comparison of technical and clinical outcomes. *J Neurointerv Surg.* 2019;32(3):97–104.

5. Jolly SS, Yusuf S, Cairns J, et al. Radial versus femoral access for coronary angiography and intervention in patients with acute coronary syndromes (RIVAL): a randomised, parallel group, multicentre trial. *Lancet.* 2011;377(9775):1409–1420.

6. Khanna O, Sweid A, Mouchtouris N, et al. Radial artery catheterization for neuroendovascular procedures. *Stroke.* 2019;50(9):2587–2590.

7. Kok MM, Weernink MGM, von Birgelen C, et al. Patient preference for radial versus femoral vascular access for elective coronary procedures: the PREVAS study. *Catheter Cardiovasc Interv.* 2018;91(1):17–24.

8. Kolkailah AA, Alreshq RS, Muhammed AM, et al. Transradial versus transfemoral approach for diagnostic coronary angiography and percutaneous coronary intervention in people with coronary artery disease. *Cochrane Database Syst Rev.* 2018;4:CD012318.

9. Mamas MA, Tosh J, Hulme W, et al. Health economic analysis of access site practice in England during changes in practice: insights from the British Cardiovascular Interventional Society. *Circ Cardiovasc Qual Outcomes.* 2018;11(5):e004482.

10. Valgimigli M, Gagnor A, Calabro P, et al. Radial versus femoral access in patients with acute coronary syndromes undergoing invasive management: a randomised multicentre trial. *Lancet.* 2015;385(9986):2465–2476.

11. Hildick-Smith DJ, Walsh JT, Lowe MD, et al. Coronary angiography in the fully anticoagulated patient: the transradial route is successful and safe. *Catheter Cardiovasc Interv.* 2003;58(1):8–10.

12. Hildick-Smith DJ, Walsh JT, Lowe MD, et al. Coronary angiography in the presence of peripheral vascular disease: femoral or brachial/radial approach? *Catheter Cardiovasc Interv.* 2000;49(1):32–37.

13. Wimmer NJ, Resnic FS, Mauri L, et al. Risk-treatment paradox in the selection of transradial access for percutaneous coronary intervention. *J Am Heart Assoc.* 2013;2(3):e000174.

14. Chen SH, Snelling BM, Sur S, et al. Transradial versus transfemoral access for anterior circulation mechanical thrombectomy: comparison of technical and clinical outcomes. *J Neurointerv Surg.* 2019;11(9):874–878.

15. Caputo RP, Simons A, Giambartolomei A, et al. Transradial cardiac catheterization in elderly patients. *Catheter Cardiovasc Interv.* 2000;51(3):287–290.

16. Shah SS, Snelling BM, Brunet MC, et al. Transradial mechanical thrombectomy for proximal middle cerebral artery occlusion in a first trimester pregnancy: case report and literature review. *World Neurosurg.* 2018;120:415–419.

17. Maud A, Khatri R, Chaudhry MRA, et al. Transradial access results in faster skin puncture to reperfusion time than transfemoral access in posterior circulation mechanical thrombectomy. *J Vasc Interv Neurol*. 2019;10(3):53–57.

18. Barria Perez AE, Costerousse O, Cieza T, et al. Feasibility and safety of early repeat transradial access within 30 days of previous coronary angiography and intervention. *Am J Cardiol*. 2017;120(8):1267–1271.

19. Dahm JB, Vogelgesang D, Hummel A, et al. A randomized trial of 5 vs. 6 French transradial percutaneous coronary interventions. *Catheter Cardiovasc Interv*. 2002;57(2):172–176.

20. Pancholy SB, Bernat I, Bertrand OF, et al. Prevention of radial artery occlusion after transradial catheterization: the PROPHET-II randomized trial. *JACC Cardiovasc Interv*. 2016;9(19):1992–1999.

21. Saito S, Ikei H, Hosokawa G, et al. Influence of the ratio between radial artery inner diameter and sheath outer diameter on radial artery flow after transradial coronary intervention. *Catheter Cardiovasc Interv*. 1999;46(2):173–178.

22. Sinha SK, Jha MJ, Mishra V, et al. Radial artery occlusion—incidence, predictors and long-term outcome after transradial catheterization: clinico-Doppler ultrasound-based study (RAIL-TRAC study). *Acta Cardiol*. 2017;72(3):318–327.

23. Abdelaal E, Molin P, Plourde G, et al. Successive transradial access for coronary procedures: experience of Quebec Heart-Lung Institute. *Am Heart J*. 2013;165(3):325–331.

24. Chen SH, Brunet MC, Sur S, et al. Feasibility of repeat transradial access for neuroendovascular procedures. *J Neurointerv Surg*. 2019;146(6):233–241.

25. Chen SH, Snelling BM, Shah SS, et al. Transradial approach for flow diversion treatment of cerebral aneurysms: a multicenter study. *J Neurointerv Surg*. 2019;150(7):322–331.

26. Kuhn AL, de Macedo Rodrigues K, Singh J, et al. Distal radial access in the anatomical snuffbox for neurointerventions: a feasibility, safety, and proof-of-concept study. *J Neurointerv Surg*. 2020;57(4):34–39.

27. Snelling BM, Sur S, Shah SS, et al. Transradial approach for complex anterior and posterior circulation interventions: technical nuances and feasibility of using current devices. *Oper Neurosurg (Hagerstown)*. 2018;66(4):443–451.

28. Barros G, Bass DI, Osbun JW, et al. Left transradial access for cerebral angiography. *J Neurointerv Surg*. 2019;32(8):227–234.

CHAPTER 6

Aneurysm Treatment

CHRISTOPHER STOREY, JONATHON LEBOVITZ, ERIC C. PETERSON, AND PASCAL M. JABBOUR

T HE GOAL OF A TRANSRADIAL ANEURYSM TREATMENT IS TO ACHIEVE the same high-quality level of embolization that would otherwise be achieved from a transfemoral route. The main limitation to aneurysm treatment from a transradial approach will be the radial artery diameter, so we must determine the amount of support required for the case. Companies are actively developing new catheters to allow for better support and trackability to improve efficiency in transradial treatments. The treatment of intracranial pathology from a transradial approach will continue to become easier.

Embolization planning should proceed as you would with any aneurysm. The first step is evaluating the size, configuration, and location of the lesion to select the best embolization method. Next, evaluate the tortuosity to determine the required support and catheter selection for the case. Posterior circulation is usually more straightforward, but anterior circulation aneurysms should be approached as you would any case that requires navigating a type 3 arch. Due to the "U-turn" the catheters must take from a transradial approach, more support is better. All techniques and systems can be utilized from a radial approach.

EQUIPMENT

Unfortunately for us neuroradialists, the innominate artery does not point at our destination as it does for cardiologists. No manufacturer has any systems designed for neurointerventional procedures from a transradial approach because, until recently, there was no need for it. The only equipment we have been able to carry over from the cardiologists is the radial sheaths.

SHORT SHEATHS

There are two main brands: Merit and Terumo. In our experience, you will become easily frustrated with the Terumo sheath because it lacks reinforcement and tends to accordion and kink. Merit sheaths are reinforced, decreasing the likelihood of kinking and making them adequate for femoral use if conversion is required. Do not try to use the Terumo radial sheath for transfemoral access because it is not reinforced and will kink. We typically use the 5 Fr Merit for diagnostics, 6 Fr Merit for biaxial construction, or start with 6 Fr or 7 Fr Merit and exchange to a 6F long sheath for increased support. The 4 Fr merit can be used with 4 Fr catheters for diagnostics as well.

As mentioned earlier, when large-caliber devices are warranted, a sheathless approach may be used. The short sheath 7 Fr Merit can be inserted without nicking the skin. Then the short sheath can be exchanged over a 0.35 Terumo wire to a 0.088 inch sheath.

LONG SHEATHS

The three best radial long sheaths that we have utilized in practice are the 6 Fr Flexor Shuttle (Cook), the 6 Fr AXS Infinity LS (Stryker), and the 6 Fr Ballast (Balt). The Infinity has a slight advantage of a bigger lumen at 0.088 inch over the 0.087 inch lumen of the Flexor Shuttle. The Neuromax (.088 inch inner diameter, 2.66 mm outer diameter) by Penumbra has essentially been abandoned for a transradial approach due to multiple difficulties with climbing and resistance. The Ballast is the best of the pack due to a slimmer distal 20 cm with a hydrophilic coating. It climbs the best, but if proximal spasm locks the catheter halfway up the common artery, it still provides enough support to deploy a pipeline with standard techniques. Also, the Ballast removes more easily for cases with spasm, recently a new catheter "RIST" was FDA approved, it is the first catheter specifically designed to access the neurovasculature through the radial approach (Figure 6.1).

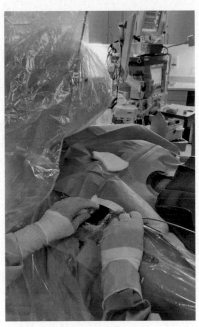

FIGURE 6.1 *Exchanging to a sheathless RIST catheter.*

The slightly larger outer diameter of the Infinity long sheath (2.76 mm) might be important to note, especially when treating patients with smaller radial arteries, as seen in women and smaller individuals. A common transradial problem is resistance due to spasm of the artery, which is directly related to the initial size of the vessel. A sheath to artery ration of <0.9 was found to be ideal from a comfort and postprocedure patency standpoint.[1]

As we treat pathologies more distally, catheter length will become a bigger issue. Using a long sheath, longer than 90 cm, will begin to cannibalize your other catheters. Sheaths that are 80 cm long are probably adequate for most individuals, but in taller and older patients with any tortuosity, the long sheath will be short of the carotid bifurcation, especially on left-sided pathology. Unless you really want distal support, in a patient with significant tortuosity, then a 100 cm sheath could be useful; otherwise we would reserve those for only stroke treatments.

DIAGNOSTIC AND SELECT CATHETERS

The Penumbra catheter in the Simmons 2 shape is best for diagnostics; there are two lengths: 120 cm and 130 cm. The Terumo Glidecatheter 4F or 5F, with a length of 100 cm, can be used, too, but not if you are planning on advancing a distal access catheter over it. If the patient has a very severe type 3 arch, then the Simmons 3 may be needed to select and image the left vertebral artery.

DISTAL ACCESS CATHETERS

Depending on the method of treatment, the set-up varies. For pipeline emboliza-tion, the Navien catheters are typically used. For a Woven Endobridge embolization, a Sophia EX is currently used. If simple coil or stent coil and the tortuosity is within reason, a 6F Envoy or 6F Benchmark can be used. Envoy and Benchmark are beneficial because they can be used through the 6F radial sheath. The Penumbra Select Simmons 5F catheter passes easily through the Benchmark (ID 0.071 inch) and Envoy (ID 0.070 inch). We find the Benchmark tracks better, but the Envoy is less expensive and works well on cases without any distal tortuosity. If you have a shaped tip, it is important that you rotate it into compliant configuration to track over the Simmons catheter. Since kinking can result, it is imperative to turn slowly and allow the torque to be transmitted throughout the length of the catheter because it can have resistance from either the ra-dial artery or the inner Simmons catheter. The inner Simmons provides support against kinking, so prior to removal make sure all the torque energy has been removed from the system and the tip is in the ideal configuration.

MICROCATHETERS AND WIRES

At this point, one should have support similar to a set-up utilizing a femoral approach. You can proceed with business as usual at this point. Any microcatheter/wire combina-tion that you prefer for aneurysm treatment can be used.

SET-UP

The key to becoming efficient with the transradial approach is a proper set-up. The hand should only be supinated about 45 degrees. This allows you to bring the arm closer to the body, which is more comfortable for the patient and works well for diagnostics as it provides access to both distal and standard transradial access. We utilize the Merit radial board, which has an accessory board that allows you to build up support for your catheters with either pads or blankets. The second benefit of keeping the arm rotated and closer to the body is that catheters aren't pointed off the bed by the trajectory of the radial artery and are instead aimed down the length of the bed. The support built up to the level of the hand provides a nice platform to work and redirects fluids medially instead of on the controls or your shoes.

ACCESS

For access, ultrasound should always be used. First, you will have less spasm and labor of radial access will be significantly decreased. The double-wall puncture technique works best with ultrasound and should decrease risk of spasm. Make sure wire passes without resistance. Any resistance encountered could result in perforation or be due to spasm. If the wire cannot be passed, then an injection through the needle can be attempted, but we usually opt for a more proximal stick.

Once the wire is safely threaded, then the hydrophilic short sheath can be passed. The radial cocktail (200 μg nitroglycerin, 5 mg cardene, and 2000 units of heparin) is then injected after verifying that the patient is not hypotensive. A road map is performed to look for a radial loop and then the wire is passed to the level of the subclavian artery and an exchange is performed for a long sheath if necessary. If not exchanging, the short sheath is double flushed and secured with a Tegaderm. We prefer to leave a syringe of heparin saline on the sheath and can flush it intermittently if any penetration of blood is noted in the sheath. If a long sheath is used, then it should be attached to a pressurized heparinized saline bag.

NUANCES

Heparinization

When treating a ruptured aneurysm, we typically only withhold the heparin portion of the cocktail if there is a fresh external ventricular drain that has been placed less than 24 hours prior to vascular access. If there is any intraparenchymal hemorrhage, we will withhold the heparin until the hemorrhage has been stable for 72 hours. We feel confident in giving 2000 units of heparin intra-arterially into the radial sheath because it does not appear to significantly alter the activated clotting time. Depending on the size of the person, we will start 4000–5000 units of heparin intravenously. We feel that only about half of the intra-arterial dose affects the activated clotting time.

Ruptured Aneurysms

Our goal for ruptured aneurysm treatment is to secure the rupture site with coils and come back later for definitive treatment if needed. This allows us to treat the ruptured aneurysm through a 6F catheter. With the 6F radial sheath that has the outer diameter of a 5F sheath, we can treat almost anyone if we can access the person's radial artery. We typically use an Envoy catheter unless there is some distal tortuosity that we feel more comfortable using a benchmark to cross. The benchmark can also help navigate any proximal tortuosity as well because the tip is more trackable.

Unruptured Aneurysm

Treatment of an unruptured aneurysm typically involves a wider range of devices and systems. The flow diversion systems can require larger and stiff catheters for deployment. It is imperative while climbing with these systems that you maintain 1:1 ration of pushing to visualized movement on fluoroscopy. As with any difficult arch from the femoral approach, any continued pushing without visualizing any movement can lead to herniation of the system. Effort to bring support as high as possible should be made. Some systems have special catheters that reduce the step-off between catheters. Stiffer wires can also provide the configurational change needed for the catheters to climb past a distal tortuosity.

VASOSPASM

Although vasospasm can be an issue with any catheter, one is more likely to encounter issues with spasm using the 6F long sheath. Anecdotally, we have noted spasm issues more commonly in women with smaller baseline radial artery size and tobacco users. To prevent a retained catheter, noting increased resistance to movement of the long sheath or catheter is paramount. Unless you are near the end of positioning the catheter, the radial approach should be aborted. Continued manipulation of a catheter or long sheath in a spastic radial artery will lead to worsening vasospasm and increased catheter fatigue, which could lead to kinking. Kinking can lead to vessel or sheath damage on removal. If catheter or long sheath remains in the subclavian or distal segment, then further verapamil can be injected. Also, a cuff can be inflated over the forearm for about 10 minutes; the tissue ischemia associated with the inflated cuff causes vasodilator release to aid in catheter removal. Patience is key. If these measures improve the vasospasm, then the catheter may be mobile only temporarily until the stimulation of removal causes further spasm and the process must be repeated. As new long sheaths and catheters come to market with proximal hydrophilic coating, this well become less of an issue.

CONCLUSION

The transradial approach for the treatment of aneurysms is safe and effective. Once support is placed where it needs to be, one can treat any aneurysm similarly to how one would treat it from a transfemoral route. Patients can have the head of the bed raised immediately after the case, which is important in patients with difficult-to-control intracranial pressure or with poor pulmonary status. Elective patients, if they are not asking for it yet, will soon be. Our aging patients with back pain cannot tolerate lying flat, which raises risk of transfemoral access. With an increased number of patients requiring treatment on anticoagulants and antiplatelets, the safety profile of the transradial approach is the leading reason to convert. To become adept at the transradial approach, one must fully commit to the approach in both interventional and diagnostic procedures.

REFERENCE

1. Gwon HC, Doh JH, Choi JH, et al. A 5Fr catheter approach reduces patient discomfort during transradial coronary intervention compared with a 6Fr approach: a prospective randomized study. *J Interv Cardiol.* 2006;19(2):141–147.

CHAPTER 7

Treatment of Arteriovenous Fistulas and Arteriovenous Malformations

NIKOLAOS MOUCHTOURIS,
OMADITYA KHANNA, ERIC C. PETERSON,
AND PASCAL M. JABBOUR

INTRODUCTION

Endovascular embolization of arteriovenous fistulas (AVFs) and arteriovenous malformations (AVMs) gained popularity over the past few decades due to the high obliteration rates achieved with low morbidity to patients. Patients with lesions in high-risk locations or with complex, deep venous drainage that were previously thought to be inoperable have fared significantly better with endovascular treatment, minimizing the risk of life-threatening intracranial hemorrhage.[1]

Depending on the angioarchitecture of the AVF/AVM, endovascular treatment can become fairly complex and challenging. Improved understanding of flow dynamics has led to the advent of multiple techniques and approaches to the treatment of such lesions.[2,3] Transarterial embolization has been the mainstay approach to the treatment of arteriovenous shunting by using acrylic glues, such as N-butylcyanoacrylate (NBCA; Codman Neurovascular, Raynham, MA), nonadhesive liquid embolic agents (Onyx; ev3, Irvine, CA), or other embolic agents, such as coils or ethyl alcohol. More recently, transvenous embolization was developed for improved nidal obliteration in lesions that are difficult to access from the arterial circulation.[4] The transvenous approach is often combined with transarterial catheterization for arterial inflow control during nidal embolization. With the development of complicated treatment strategies, navigating an increasing number of catheters of varying sizes and lengths as well as simultaneous deployment of embolic agents and devices, endovascular treatment of AVF/AVMs has been become a fascinating but challenging undertaking.

Adoption of Transradial Catheterization for Endovascular Treatment

While femoral artery catheterization has been used historically for cerebral angiography, the recent adoption of the transradial approach has also been utilized for the treatment of AVF/AVM with great success. The equipment necessary for embolization includes microcatheters, balloon-tipped microcatheters, distal access agents, and embolic agents. Microcatheter options include either over the wire, such as the Echelon (eV3 Neurovascular Irvine, CA), or flow directed, such as the Marathon (ev3, Irvine, CA) and Magic (Balt, Montmorency, France). The most commonly used balloon catheter include the Scepter balloon (MicroVention, Tustin, CA), and embolic agents include Onyx (ev3, Irvine, CA) or n-butyl cyanoacrylate (nBCA; Codman Neurovascular, Raynham, MA). Distal access catheters are advanced in the anterior, middle, or posterior cerebral arteries and utilized so that the microcatheter is advanced into the AVM without traversing a long distance. All of these can be deployed with ease via the radial access route. The proximity of the radial artery to the cerebral vasculature is an added benefit when navigating a number of catheters through the fragile, abnormal arteriovenous vasculature. Even in transvenous cases more and more the cephalic vein in the upper extremity is being accessed, then a catheter is being navigated to the internal jugular vein.

Biaxial versus Triaxial Set-up

Depending on the need for biaxial versus triaxial support, a different set of sheaths and catheters are used. Following are the most commonly used set-ups:

Triaxial:

1. Sheathless 6/5 Fr shuttle sheath (Cook) versus Ballast long sheath (Balt) versus a 6/5 Fr Fubuki long sheath (Asahi) versus AXS Infinity long sheath (Stryker)
2. Intermediate catheter
3. Microcatheter/balloon microcatheter

Biaxial:

1. 6 Fr radial sheath Prelude Merit versus Slender Terumo
2. Intermediate catheter
3. Microcatheter/balloon microcatheter

The Transradial Catheterization Technique

Ultrasound-guided catheterization of the radial artery is performed using a 6 Fr sheath (Prelude or Slender). An intra-arterial cocktail of 200 μg of nitroglycerin, 5 mg of nicardipine, and 2000 Units of heparin is given through the sheath and a road map is performed.[5] If the plan is for a triaxial setup, exchange is performed with a 035 Terumo guide wire to the long sheath Shuttle/Ballast/Fubuki/Infinity (or another long sheath); then a Simmons 2 Penumbra catheter is inserted inside the long sheath. It is shaped in the arch and the vessel of interest is catheterized with the Simmons 2. The long sheath is then advanced over the Simmons 2, the Simmons 2 is removed, and an intermediate catheter is inserted and advanced distally. Lastly, the microcatheter is advanced to the lesion and the embolization is performed.

Transradial Catheterization for Intraoperative Angiography

Transradial catheterization is also beneficial for patients who undergo microsurgical resection and require intraoperative cerebral angiography.[6] Arterial access can be challenging depending on the positioning required for the resection of the AVF/AVM. Patients undergo radial artery catheterization for blood pressure monitoring intraoperatively, which can then be converted into the access route for the intraoperative angiogram. This access route is feasible even in lateral or prone positioning without any limitations. In a study by Osbun et al., 27 patients underwent intraoperative transradial cerebral angiography after microsurgical treatment of AVM, AVF, and aneurysms with two patients having to be converted to femoral catheterization. In that same study, six patients had to undergo follow-up cerebral angiography and the same access site was successfully used in five of them, while one was found to have asymptomatic radial artery occlusion; the femoral artery had to be catheterized instead.[6] Chalouhi et al. reported a series of 10 patients undergoing transradial intraoperative angiography with an average time of 9.3 minutes.[7] None of the patients required to be converted to transfemoral catheterization and no access or thromboembolic complications were seen.[7] Furthermore, patients often undergo preoperative endovascular embolization the day prior to microsurgery, and the access sheath can be utilized the following day for the intraoperative angiography without any mobility restraints.[8] Depending on the operative positioning, left transradial catheterization is also an option and it has been utilized for AVM embolization.[9] Lastly, transradial catheterization allows for early mobilization postoperatively regardless of when the access sheath is removed.[5]

CASE ILLUSTRATION

A 64-year-old female who presented with 5 days of headaches was found on noncontrast head computerized tomography (CT) to have intraventricular hemorrhage in the right lateral ventricle, and CT angiogram showed a 2.4 × 0.7 × 0.7 cm AVM adjacent to the septum pellucidum. The following day she underwent a cerebral angiogram via right radial artery catheterization. A 5 French sheath was placed in the right radial artery. A cocktail of heparin, nitroglycerin, and nicardipine was administered to avoid vasospasm. A six-vessel angiogram was performed demonstrating the AVM being filled from the right A2 and medial posterior choroidal feeding arteries. The AVM drained into the internal cerebral veins and vein of Galen (Figures 7.1, 7.2, 7.3, and 7.4). After a lengthy discussion, the decision was to proceed with combined transarterial and transvenous embolization. The right radial sheath from the diagnostic angiogram was exchanged for a 6 French sheath. 6 French sheaths were inserted in the right common femoral artery and the left internal jugular vein. Two Scepter XC balloons were advanced into the A1-2 junction and the right posterior choroidal artery.

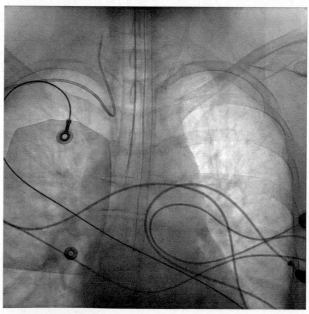

FIGURE 7.1 *Arterial and venous access.*

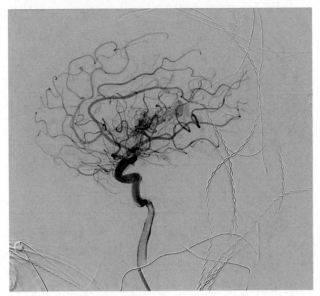

FIGURE 7.2 *Lateral view showing the AVM.*

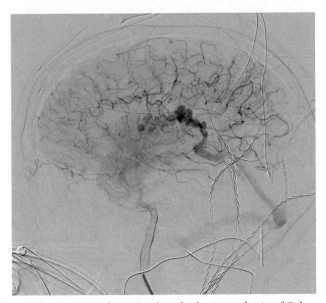

FIGURE 7.3 *Venous drainage into the internal cerebral veins and vein of Galen.*

A Navien 072 was advanced from the left IJ sheath 6 French sheath into the distal straight sinus. Using an Echelon catheter, a coil was deployed in the internal cerebral vein, but not detached. The two balloons were inflated, and all arterial inflow into the AVM was suspended; 8 cc of Onyx 18 was injected from the transvenous catheter into the AVM nidus. An additional 0.2 cc of Onyx was injected from the A2 perforator. A final angiographic run was performed showing complete exclusion of the AVM from the circulation (Figures 7.5, 7.6, and 7.7).

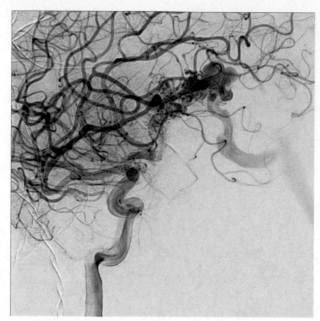

FIGURE 7.4 *View of the nidus.*

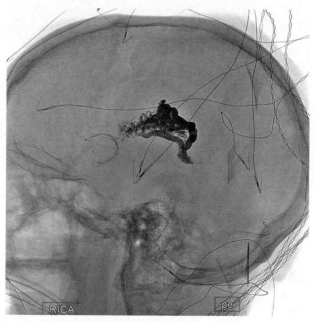

FIGURE 7.5 *The onyx cast on a lateral view.*

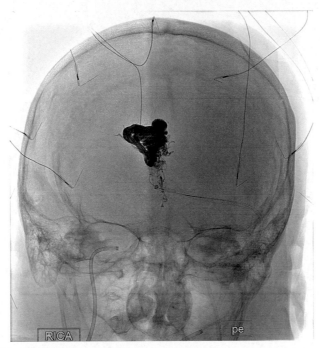

FIGURE 7.6 *The onyx cast on an AP view.*

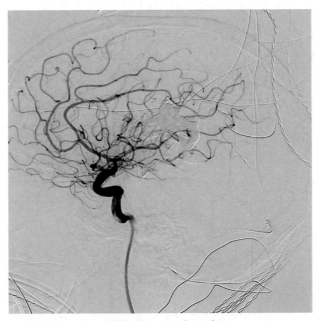

FIGURE 7.7 *Complete obliteration of the AVM on a lateral view.*

REFERENCES

1. Subat YW, Dasenbrock HH, Gross BA, et al. Periprocedural intracranial hemorrhage after embolization of cerebral arteriovenous malformations: a meta-analysis. *J Neurosurg.* 2019:1–11. doi:10.3171/ 2019.5.JNS183204.

2. Zaki Ghali MG, Kan P, Britz GW. Curative embolization of arteriovenous malformations. *World Neurosurg.* 2019;129:467–486.

3. Iosif C, Mendes GA, Saleme S, et al. Endovascular transvenous cure for ruptured brain arteriovenous malformations in complex cases with high Spetzler-Martin grades. *J Neurosurg.* 2015;122(5):1229–1238. doi:10.3171/2014.9.JNS141714.

4. Chen CJ, Norat P, Ding D, et al. Transvenous embolization of brain arteriovenous malformations: a review of techniques, indications, and outcomes. *Neurosurg Focus.* 2018;45(1):E13. doi:10.3171/ 2018.3.FOCUS18113.

5. Khanna O, Sweid A, Mouchtouris N, et al. Radial artery catheterization for neuroendovascular procedures. *Stroke.* 2019;50(9):2587–2590. doi:10.1161/STROKEAHA.119.025811.

6. Osbun JW, Patel B, Levitt MR, et al. Transradial intraoperative cerebral angiography: a multicenter case series and technical report. *J Neurointerv Surg.* 2020;12(2):170–175. doi:10.1136/ neurintsurg-2019-015207.

7. Chalouhi N, Sweid A, Al Saiegh F, et al. Initial experience with transradial intraoperative angiography in aneurysm clipping: technique, feasibility, and case series. *World Neurosurg.* 2020;134:e554–e558. doi:10.1016/j.wneu.2019.10.130.

8. Yoon W, Kim H, Kim YW, Kim SR, Park IS. Usefulness and stability of intraoperative digital subtraction angiography using the transradial route in arteriovenous malformation surgery. *World Neurosurg.* 2018;111:e799–e805.

9. Barros G, Bass DI, Osbun JW, et al. Left transradial access for cerebral angiography. *J Neurointerv Surg.* 2020;12(4):427–430. doi:10.1136/neurintsurg-2019-015386.

CHAPTER 8

Carotid Stenting

OMADITYA KHANNA, NIKOLAOS
MOUCHTOURIS, ERIC C. PETERSON, AND
PASCAL M. JABBOUR

INTRODUCTION

Carotid artery stenosis (CAS) is caused by progressive deposition of atheromatous plaques in the extracranial carotid artery, most pronounced at the carotid bifurcation. The progressive narrowing of the proximal internal carotid artery causes turbulent flow, leading to shearing forces against the luminal wall of the vessel, with resultant endothelial inflammation. Rupture of plaque at the carotid bifurcation can embolize distally to the intracranial vessels, causing an ischemic infarct of the territory supplied by the occluded vessel. Indeed, CAS accounts for one-third of all strokes in the United States.[1] Medical comorbidities such as obesity, tobacco use, and diabetes mellitus have been shown to accelerate the progression of carotid artery disease.

In the Carotid Revascularization Endarterectomy versus Stenting Trial (CREST), the outcomes of patients with carotid stenosis treated with carotid endarterectomy were compared with those treated with carotid artery stenting. Patients with symptomatic stenosis (>50% in severity) and asymptomatic stenosis (>60% in severity) were included in the trial. The trial showed similar rates of perioperative events and mortality rates between the two groups, and equivalent low rates of restenosis or occlusion.[2] Furthermore, the Stenting and Angioplasty with Protection in Patients at High Risk for Endarterectomy (SAPPHIRE) trial also lent further credence to the treatment paradigm that patients who are medically high-risk should preferentially be treated endovascularly via carotid artery stent.

Radial access is a reasonable alternative over the femoral approach for CAS, especially in patients with extensive peripheral vascular disease and patients with anatomical variations (aortic arch II–III or bovine arch). Bovine type aortic arch, which has an incidence of 11%–29%, makes it very challenging for stenting left internal carotid pathology using a femoral approach.[3] In addition, bovine aortic arch may be associated with type III aortic arch, and elongated type II and III aortic arch constitute another challenge for transfemoral access. The radial approach is associated with low morbidity, mortality benefit, lower hospital stay, and cost reduction. The randomized RADial access for CARotid artery stenting (RADCAR) study found that transradial access for CAS safe and efficacious. The major access-site complications and major cardiac and cerebral events were 0.9%. The crossover rate was higher compared to transfemoral route access (10% vs 1.5%); however, the length of hospital stay was shorter in the transradial group. It has been well described and broadly accepted that there is a learning curve to achieve optimal outcomes with the transradial approach. Operators embracing the radial access for CAS need to take that into consideration and be vigilant to maintain the safety profile of the approach.

ANATOMIC CONSIDERATIONS

Aortic Arch Morphology

The origin level of the great vessels off the aortic arch characterize three types of arches (I–III). Vessels originating from the same or above the horizontal plane traversing the outer curvature of the aortic arch are type I. The innominate originating between the two planes originating from outer and inner curvature of the aortic arch are type II. While type III, the innominate artery originates below a plane traversing the inner curvature of the aortic arch. The more inferior the origin is, the more likely it is to selectively catheterize the vessels.

Carotid Artery Morphology

The tortuosity and the atherosclerosis burden of the carotid artery increase complexity and affect the deliverability of the diagnostic catheter. An angle ≥ 60 between the internal carotid artery and common carotid artery increases the relative risk of death and stroke after CAS by ~5 times.[4]

PREPROCEDURAL PLANNING

Preprocedural imaging, whether computed tomography angiography (CTA) or magnetic resonance angiography (MRA), is essential for optimal outcomes. Findings such as atherosclerotic and calcific disease, arch anomalies, and unfavorable anatomy (acute angles of <50 degrees) are essential to know for more accurate risk assessment and to lower the incidence of crossover. For example, knowing that a patient with a left internal carotid artery stenosis has a type 1 aortic arch with an acute take off of the internal artery gives an idea that the success rate is only 40%–50%.[5] Folmar et al. noted successful CAS outcomes in 97% of right pathology, 80% of bovine pathology, and only 54% of left pathology.[5] Patients with a severe angle between the right subclavian artery and the right common carotid artery may benefit from a left radial access.[6]

TECHNIQUE

Multiple factors are taken into consideration when choosing the optimal technique for transradial CAS. Mainly the vascular tortuosity and aortic arch morphology delineates how much proximal support is needed, and the stent size stratified into ≤8 mm or >8 mm. Access may be achieved using two different platforms, either a sheath-based system or a sheathless-based platform. The decision regarding which approach should be used is based on the vascular tortuosity and the need for proximal support, and the size of the stent. When proximal support is required and a stent size more than 8 mm is used, then a sheathless approach should be used. If no extra support is needed and a stent 8 mm or smaller is used, a 6 Fr prelude sheath is inserted. A coaxial system of a 6F guide catheter (Benchmark, Envoy) and a 5F diagnostic catheter (Penumbra Sim select or Berenstein select) over a 0.038 glide wire are advanced into the aortic arch, the Simmons 2 is shaped and the vessel of interest is catheterized, and the 6 Fr guide is advanced on top of the Simmons 2.

When proximal support is needed, then a sheathless approach should be used. A short sheath 7 Fr Merit can be inserted without nicking the skin. Then the short sheath can be exchanged with a 0.35 Terumo glide wire, and a 6 Fr long sheath is inserted (Ballast 0.088 inch, Flexor shuttle, AXS Infinity LS). Then a 5 Fr diagnostic catheter is inserted into the long sheath (Simmons 2 catheter, Berenstein select) and advanced under road map into the aortic arch. The advantage of the sheathless technique is that the long sheath is advanced into the common carotid artery and left in place for the entire procedure; the procedure can be done with only the long sheath or a 6 Fr guide catheter (benchmark/6Envoy) is inserted inside the long sheath. This technique minimizes the number of catheter and wire exchanges, dropping the risk of thrombus dislodgement. The drawback is that the guiding sheath may herniate while deploying the stent unless it is advanced far enough into the common carotid artery.

Common Carotid Artery Access

After achieving access into the aortic arch, selecting the common carotid artery may be technically challenging. Two techniques that may be used to overcome such a hurdle are the wire-exchanging technique, or a catheter reformation and retrograde advancement. The reformation of the diagnostic catheter is performed either in the ascending aorta or the descending aorta or by deflexion of the 0.038 glide wire over the aortic valve. The tip of the diagnostic catheter is manipulated to guide the catheter into either the left common carotid artery or the right common carotid artery. The 0.038 glide wire is first advanced into the common carotid artery followed by advancing the diagnostic catheter.

After achieving access into the common carotid artery, the rest of the procedure is completed by advancing the long sheath or guide catheter on top of the Simmons 2.

CASE ILLUSTRATION

The patient is a 70-year-old male with a history of atrial fibrillation, who presented for evaluation of right eye amaurosis fugax. An MRA did not reveal any intracranial infarct. A CTA was performed that showed high-grade (80%) stenosis of the right internal carotid artery. The patient had the plaque high-riding; therefore, the decision was made to proceed with placement of a carotid artery stent (see Figure 8.1).

The patient was identified on the INR table. The right wrist was prepped and draped, and local lidocaine is administered. Radial artery catheterization was achieved using ultrasound guidance, via double-wall puncture and Seldinger technique. After access is achieved with a 6 Fr prelude sheath, the intra-arterial cocktail of 5 mg of Cardene, 200 μg of nitroglycerin, and 200 Units of heparin was given. Then a radial run was performed and under road map a 035 Terumo glide wire and a Simmons 2 Penumbra inside a benchmark were advanced to the arch, the Simmons 2 was shaped and the right internal carotid artery was catheterized, and the Benchmark was advanced in the common carotid artery on the right.

Next, anteroposterior and lateral cranial cervical runs were obtained, which delineate the degree of carotid stenosis and morphology of the luminal plaque. Next, a 5 mm spider distal protection device was navigated into the internal carotid artery distal to the area of stenosis. At this time, a balloon angioplasty was performed. Then a stent was deployed.

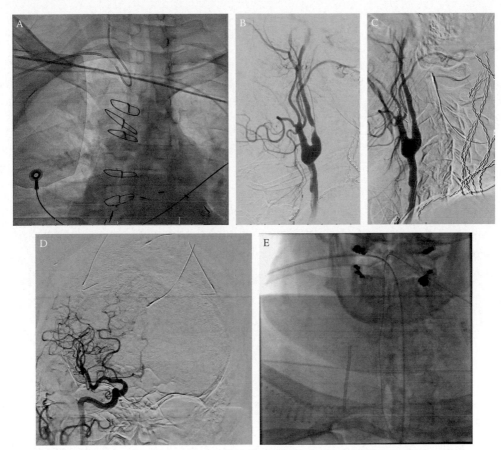

FIGURE 8.1 *Right radial access is obtained. A fluoroscopy shot showing the Simmons 2 catheter engaged in the common carotid artery on the right side and proximal to it the Benchmark catheter (A). A lateral cervical run is performed, which shows severe stenosis of the right internal carotid artery (ICA) just distal to its origin at the bifurcation (B). A carotid artery stent is placed, with interval improvement of the degree of stenosis (C). A cranial run using a right ICA injection is obtained which shows patency of the intracranial vessels, without any evidence of thromboembolism after deployment of the stent (D). Benchmark from radial to right common artery (E).*

Another cervical run was performed to confirm resolution of the stenosis, and a cranial run is evaluated to ensure no distal thromboembolism has occurred after stent placement. Once satisfied, the catheters are sequentially removed.

After the procedure is complete, the sheath is removed and a radial artery compression device (TR Band, Terumo Interventional Systems) is applied. The compression band is inflated with air, and it is slowly, sequentially deflated after 1 hour according to protocol.

CONCLUSION

Currently, radial artery catheterization is the preferred method of access for cardiac interventionalists, and several large-scale randomized, controlled studies have shown that it is safe and effective.[7] Femoral artery catheterization requires patients to tolerate an uncomfortable procedure, with associated potential complications such as pseudoaneurysm formation, retroperitoneal hematoma, arteriovenous fistula, and artery occlusion.[8–10] Several large-scale, multicenter trials and case series have shown that radial artery access is associated with fewer access-site complications than the standard transfemoral approach, with better patient satisfaction measures.[11–13]

Currently, radial artery access is scarcely used for neuroendovascular procedures, but it is starting to gain more widespread use.[14–16] At our institution, we have transitioned our practice toward performing the majority of our neuroendovascular procedures via a transradial approach, and we have recently published our case series that demonstrates its feasibility.[1] The use of radial artery catheterization confers a technically favorable alternative to navigate tortuous aortic arches and neck vasculature. Once the desired internal carotid artery has been catheterized, balloon angioplasty and stent placement can be performed in a similar fashion as transfemoral access.

REFERENCES

1. Yamazaki M, Uchiyama S. Pathophysiology of carotid stenosis. *Brain Nerve.* 2010;62(12):1269–1275.
2. Brott TG, Hobson RW, 2nd, Howard G, et al. Stenting versus endarterectomy for treatment of carotid-artery stenosis. *N Engl J Med.* 2010;363(1):11–23.
3. Malone C, Urbania T, Crook S, Hope M. Bovine aortic arch: a novel association with thoracic aortic dilation. *Clin Radiol.* 2012;67(1):28–31.
4. Naggara O, Touzé E, Beyssen B, et al. Anatomical and technical factors associated with stroke or death during carotid angioplasty and stenting: results from the endarterectomy versus angioplasty in patients with symptomatic severe carotid stenosis (EVA-3S) trial and systematic review. *Stroke.* 2011;42(2):380–388.
5. Folmar J, Sachar R, Mann T. Transradial approach for carotid artery stenting: a feasibility study. *Catheter Cardiovasc Interv.* 2007;69(3):355–361.
6. Patel T, Shah S, Ranjan A, Malhotra H, Pancholy S, Coppola J. Contralateral transradial approach for carotid artery stenting: a feasibility study. *Catheter Cardiovasc Interv.* 2010;75(2):268–275.
7. Ibanez B, James S, Agewall S, et al. 2017 ESC Guidelines for the management of acute myocardial infarction in patients presenting with ST-segment elevation: The Task Force for the management of acute myocardial infarction in patients presenting with ST-segment elevation of the European Society of Cardiology (ESC). *Eur Heart J.* 2018;39(2):119–177.
8. Tavakol M, Ashraf S, Brener SJ. Risks and complications of coronary angiography: a comprehensive review. *Glob J Health Sci.* 2012;4(1):65–93.
9. Fifi JT, Meyers PM, Lavine SD, et al. Complications of modern diagnostic cerebral angiography in an academic medical center. *J Vasc Interv Radiol.* 2009;20(4):442–447.
10. Hibbert B, Simard T, Wilson KR, et al. Transradial versus transfemoral artery approach for coronary angiography and percutaneous coronary intervention in the extremely obese. *JACC Cardiovasc Interv.* 2012;5(8):819–826.
11. Jolly SS, Yusuf S, Cairns J, et al. Radial versus femoral access for coronary angiography and intervention in patients with acute coronary syndromes (RIVAL): a randomised, parallel group, multicentre trial. *Lancet.* 2011;377(9775):1409–1420.
12. Ando G, Capodanno D. Radial versus femoral access in invasively managed patients with acute coronary syndrome: a systematic review and meta-analysis. *Ann Intern Med.* 2015;163(12):932–940.

13. Mehta SR, Jolly SS, Cairns J, et al. Effects of radial versus femoral artery access in patients with acute coronary syndromes with or without ST-segment elevation. *J Am Coll Cardiol.* 2012;60(24):2490–2499.

14. Snelling BM, Sur S, Shah SS, et al. Transradial cerebral angiography: techniques and outcomes. *J Neurointerv Surg.* 2018;10(9):874–881.

15. Chen SH, Snelling BM, Sur S, et al. Transradial versus transfemoral access for anterior circulation mechanical thrombectomy: comparison of technical and clinical outcomes. *J Neurointerv Surg.* 2019;11(9):874–878. doi:10.1136/neurintsurg-2018-014485.

16. Levy EI, Boulos AS, Fessler RD, et al. Transradial cerebral angiography: an alternative route. *Neurosurgery.* 2002;51(2):335–340;discussion 340–332.

CHAPTER 9

Transradial Approach for Stroke

STEPHANIE H. CHEN, PASCAL M. JABBOUR, AND ERIC C. PETERSON

INTRODUCTION

Mechanical thrombectomy (MT) is the standard of care for patients presenting with acute large-vessel occlusion ischemic stroke (LVOS).[1] While the transfemoral approach (TFA) was predominantly used in the MT trials, several studies have demonstrated that complex aortic arch and carotid arterial anatomy are associated with increased technical difficulty and thus prolonged procedural times and complication rates.[1-3] Specifically in MT, complex aortic arch anatomy and internal carotid artery (ICA) tortuosity as assessed by the B.A.D. vessel score was associated with significant increases in puncture to reperfusion times.[4] The transradial approach (TRA) confers a technically favorable trajectory in cases of torturous arch and neck vasculature.[5] Furthermore, TRA is increasingly the preferred approach for all neurointerventional procedures due to multiple studies demonstrating a significant decrease in vascular site complications as well as overwhelming patient preference.[6-11]

PATIENT SELECTION

A primary transradial approach is used for all posterior circulation LVOS. The direct anatomy of the vertebral artery from the subclavian artery allows for significantly shorter puncture to recanalization time in posterior circulation strokes (29.2 ± 17.6 minutes in the transradial group vs. 63.9 ± 56.7 minutes in the transfemoral group).[12] Typically a right radial approach is preferred if the right vertebral artery is dominant or the vertebral arteries are codominant. If the left vertebral artery is dominant, left distal radial artery access in the anatomical snuffbox is often used because the arm can be draped across the body, improving the ergonomics of the procedure.

Insert Figure 9.5 HereAll acute stroke patients at our institution undergo a computed tomography angiogram (CTA) of the head and neck, including the aortic arch. For anterior circulation LVOS, a primary transradial approach is used if the CTA demonstrates a bovine arch variant, aortic arch type II, or aortic arch type III.[5] In our initial experience, we found similar recanalization times between TRA and TFA in patients with challenging vascular anatomy undergoing MT. However, with more experience, efficiency, and equipment improvements, we anticipate improved outcomes and gradual transition to default radial for all neurointerventional procedures. Finally, we also consider primary TRA for MT in patients with large body habitus, previous iliac stenting or bypass, femoral occlusion, or who are on antiplatelet and anticoagulation medications.

TECHNIQUE

Radial Artery Access

The right radial artery is used for MT of the anterior circulation or for posterior circulation LVOS from the right vertebral artery. The left radial or distal radial artery is used in cases of posterior circulation LVOS with a left dominant vertebral artery. Procedural

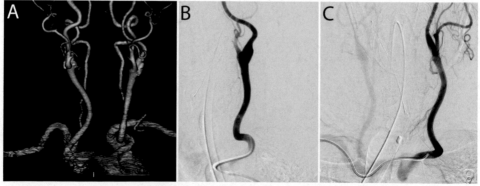

FIGURE 9.1 *(A) Computed tomography angiography reconstruction demonstrating a bovine arch anatomic variant where the innominate artery and left common carotid artery share a common origin from the aortic arch. (B) Digital subtraction angiography (DSA) of left common carotid artery catheterization of a bovine arch from a femoral approach. (C) DSA demonstrating more favorable trajectory of left common carotid artery catheterization of a bovine arch from the radial approach.*

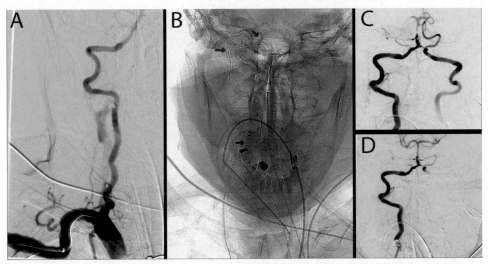

FIGURE 9.2 *An 89-year-old female with a past medical history of atrial fibrillation on apixaban who presented with sudden onset left hemiparesis 2 hours prior and a National Institute of Health Stroke Scale score of 17 on arrival. Computed tomography angiography demonstrated basilar occlusion and she was taken for mechanical thrombectomy. (A) Digital subtraction angiography (DSA) demonstrating trajectory from right radial artery approach to the right vertebral artery. (B) The Solumbra technique was performed with an 0.088 inch Infinity guide catheter (black arrow), 0.068 inch aspiration catheter (red arrow), 0.027 inch microcatheter, and a 6 mm × 40 mm stentriever (blue arrow). (C) DSA after three passes with the stentriever with evidence of residual basilar stenosis. (D) DSA of right vertebral artery after a 2 mm × 15 mm noncompliant balloon was telescoped through the aspiration and guide catheter across the stenosis and a submaximal angioplasty was performed.*

details for obtaining transradial access can be found in Chapter 2. Specifically for MT, a 6 or 7 French transradial introducer sheath (Glidesheath Slender, Terumo, Somerset, NJ) is placed. The prophylactic spasmolytic agents (2.5 mg verapamil; 200 µg nitroglycerin) are administered; however, unlike other TRA neurointerventions, prophylactic intravenous heparin to prevent radial artery occlusion is not given in MT, due to the potentially devastating risks of hemorrhagic conversion after stroke as compared to clinically insignificant and low radial artery occlusion rates (4%).[13] However, many operators give heparin routinely in TFA MT, and those that are facile with TRA also give heparin for their MT cases when performed via TRA. In our lab, in the rare event of a prolonged MT case exceeding 1 hour, we administer 3000 Units of heparin to prevent clot formation on the guide in the arm.

Catheter Selection

Currently, we prefer to use a 0.088 inch Infinity guide catheter system (Stryker Neurovascular, Kalamazoo, MI) for TRA mechanical thrombectomy. Access is obtained and a 7 Fr Glidesheath Slender (Terumo, Somerset, NJ) is inserted into the radial artery.

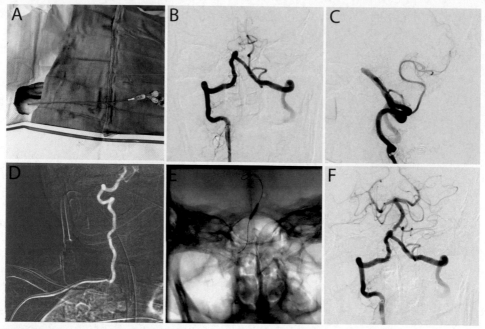

FIGURE 9.3 *A 66-year-old male with a history of ischemic stroke presented after waking up with nausea, vomiting, and speech disturbances 6 hours prior; found to have a National Institute of Health Stroke Scale of 7 on arrival. A computed tomography angiography demonstrated a basilar occlusion and patient was taken emergently for mechanical thrombectomy. A right radial approach was selected due to codominant vertebral arteries and (A) an 0.088 inch guide catheter was placed sheathless in the radial artery. (B) Anteroposterior and (C) lateral digital subtraction angiography (DSA) demonstrating complete basilar occlusion. (D) A 0.088 inch guide system with a 0.068 inch aspiration catheter, 0.027 inch microcatheter, and 4 mm × 40 mm stentriever was navigated into the right vertebral artery from a right radial approach. (C) Submaximal angioplasty of an area of residual stenosis was then performed with a noncompliant 2 mm × 9 mm noncompliant balloon. (D) DSA demonstrating complete reperfusion.*

The antispasmodics and radial artery angiogram are performed. If the anatomy is appropriate (without radial artery anomalies), the 7 Fr glidesheath is then exchanged over a 0.035 inch guide wire for the 0.088 inch Infinity guide catheter with the stylet, which is placed sheathless into the radial artery. The catheter is advanced over the wire into the subclavian artery, where the stylet and wire are then removed. A 125 cm Simmons 2 Select catheter (Penumbra, Alameda, CA) is navigated over a guide wire into the target ICA. A 125 Berenstein Select catheter is used for vertebral artery (VA) catheterization from the subclavian artery. The guide catheter is tracked over the Select catheter, and the remainder of the mechanical thrombectomy is performed in identical fashion to TFA with either "Solumbra" technique or first-pass aspiration alone.

The 0.088 inch guide catheter is preferable due to its large inner diameter, which provides sufficient space for all modern aspiration catheters as well as sufficient support to advance the aspiration catheter and stentrievers. However, in cases of posterior circulation

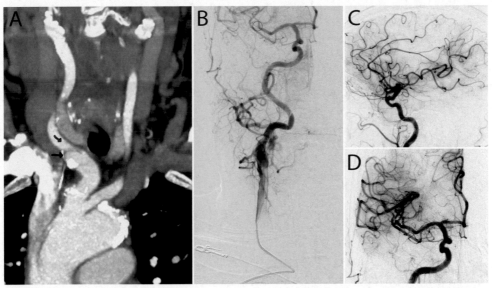

FIGURE 9.4 *A 72-year-old female with a history of coronary artery disease and deep venous thrombosis on apixaban who developed acute onset of confusion and aphasia 10 hours prior with a National Institute of Health Stroke Scale of 14 on arrival. She was found to have a right M2 occlusion on computed tomography angiography (CTA) with a significant perfusion mismatch on computed tomography perfusion. The patient had a heavily calcified femoral artery and decision was made to proceed transradial. (A) Coronal CTA of the neck demonstrating acute angle between right subclavian artery (black arrow) and right common carotid artery (blue arrow). (B) Catheterization and digital subtraction angiography (DSA) of the right internal carotid artery with Simmons 2 Select catheter from right transradial approach showing trajectory as well as the inferior division M2 occlusion (red circle). Postthrombectomy (C) lateral and (D) anteroposterior DSA of the right internal carotid artery demonstrating partial reperfusion.*

occlusions where the vertebral artery is smaller *or* in the case of very small radial arteries, a 6 French system can be used instead. We prefer a 6 Fr Benchmark (Penumbra, Alameda, CA) or Envoy DA guide catheter (Codman Neuro, Raynham, MA). In these cases, a 6 French vascular sheath is inserted into the radial artery, and the guide catheters are coaxially navigated into distal ICA/VA over a 125 cm Simmons 2/Berenstein Select diagnostic catheter (Penumbra, Alameda, CA). Subsequently, the stentriever is then deployed using standard procedure and retrieved with manual aspiration of the guide catheter.

For balloon guide catheter plus stentriever techniques, a 5 Fr Simmons 2 catheter is introduced into a 6F or 7F sheath and used to navigate to the target ICA. Over an exchange length guidewire, the sheath and catheter are removed, and a 6 or 7F Cello balloon guide (Medtronic, Irvine, CA) is brought into the ICA. Thereafter, the stentriever is deployed using standard procedure and retrieved with the balloon inflated and manual aspiration from the guide catheter. We find this method time-consuming and cumbersome; thus, it is not preferred with the currently available catheters (Figures 9.1–9.5).

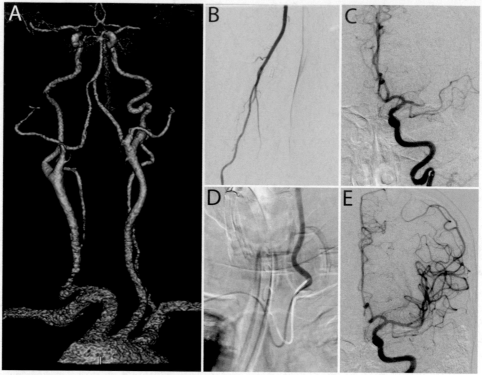

FIGURE 9.5 *A 51-year-old morbidly obese male with a history of deep venous thrombosis on apixaban presented to the emergency room after waking up with confusion and right upper-extremity weakness, with a National Institute of Health Stroke Scale of 9 on arrival. (A) Computed tomography angiography 3D reconstruction demonstrates a type I aortic arch and left M1 occlusion. Decision was made to proceed with the transradial approach due to large body habitus and anticoagulation use. (B) Radial artery angiogram shows a normal brachial artery bifurcation. (C) Initial LICA digital subtraction angiography (DSA) with left M1 occlusion. (D) Catheterization and DSA of the left common carotid artery from transradial approach with a Simmons 2 catheter. (E) Complete reperfusion on post-thrombectomy DSA after one pass with 4 mm × 40 mm stentriever, 0.068 inch aspiration catheter, and 0.088 inch guide.*

At this time, catheter and device selection for mechanical thrombectomy is limited for the transradial approach. A 6F and 7F system limits use of larger balloon guide catheters. Furthermore, access catheters and guide systems have been designed for TFA primarily, and there are no commercially available systems designed specifically for navigating the cervical and cranial vasculature via TRA at this time. With the advent of newer devices and technology, there is great potential for taking better advantage of the anatomical configuration of the great vessels approached via the right or left subclavian artery. At present, the operator should be aware that using femoral nonhydrophillically coated guides without a sheath risks vasospasm. If spasm is encountered during an MT TRA, usually the guide is unable to be advanced into the ICA. Usually an aspiration catheter can still be advanced into the M1 and the thrombectomy can be performed with either direct aspiration or Solumbra techniques. If not, however, conversion to TFA (if possible) should be considered and the stuck guide catheter managed as outlined in Chapter 10.

REFERENCES

1. Goyal M et al. Endovascular thrombectomy after large-vessel ischaemic stroke: a meta-analysis of individual patient data from five randomised trials. *Lancet.* 2016;387(10029):1723–1731.
2. Togay-Isikay C et al. Carotid artery tortuosity, kinking, coiling: stroke risk factor, marker, or curiosity? *Acta Neurol Belg.* 2005;105(2):68–72.
3. Maus V et al. Maximizing first-pass complete reperfusion with SAVE. *Clin Neuroradiol.* 2018;28(3):327–338.
4. Snelling BM et al. Unfavorable vascular anatomy is associated with increased revascularization time and worse outcome in anterior circulation thrombectomy. *World Neurosurg.* 2018;120:e976–e983.
5. Chen SH et al. Transradial versus transfemoral access for anterior circulation mechanical thrombectomy: comparison of technical and clinical outcomes. *J Neurointerv Surg.* 2019;109(7):132–141.
6. Mamas MA et al. Health economic analysis of access site practice in England during changes in practice: insights from the British Cardiovascular Interventional Society. *Circ Cardiovasc Qual Outcomes.* 2018;11(5):e004482.
7. Kolkailah AA et al. Transradial versus transfemoral approach for diagnostic coronary angiography and percutaneous coronary intervention in people with coronary artery disease. *Cochrane Database Syst Rev.* 2018;4:CD012318.
8. Kok MM et al. Patient preference for radial versus femoral vascular access for elective coronary procedures: the PREVAS study. *Catheter Cardiovasc Interv.* 2018;91(1):17–24.
9. Khanna O et al. Radial artery catheterization for neuroendovascular procedures. *Stroke.* 2019;50(9):2587–2590.
10. Jolly SS et al. Radial versus femoral access for coronary angiography and intervention in patients with acute coronary syndromes (RIVAL): a randomised, parallel group, multicentre trial. *Lancet.* 2011;377(9775):1409–1420.
11. Jolly SS et al. Radial versus femoral access for coronary angiography or intervention and the impact on major bleeding and ischemic events: a systematic review and meta-analysis of randomized trials. *Am Heart J.* 2009;157(1):132–140.
12. Maud A et al. Transradial access results in faster skin puncture to reperfusion time than transfemoral access in posterior circulation mechanical thrombectomy. *J Vasc Interv Neurol.* 2019;10(3):53–57.
13. Pancholy SB et al. Prevention of radial artery occlusion after transradial catheterization: the PROPHET-II randomized trial. *JACC Cardiovasc Interv.* 2016;9(19):1992–1999.

CHAPTER 10

Left Transradial Approach

AHMAD SWEID, ERIC C. PETERSON, AND
PASCAL M. JABBOUR

CEREBRAL TRANSRADIAL ANGIOGRAPHIES ARE EXCLUSIVELY PERFORMED using the right side, except for isolated left vertebral artery pathology or certain anatomical variations.[1] Left radial access is an essential adjunct that can be used as a bailout when the right access fails or when the target vessel may be reached from the left side to alternate between right and left radial artery access. The left radial artery has certain advantages and limitations that operators should be aware of.

First, the left transradial approach allows for the use of the nondominant hand in the majority of patients and thereby allows the wrist to heal with fewer restrictions in daily activities. In addition, using the snuffbox in the left radial side allows more ergonomic left-hand positioning over the groin and obviates the need for hand supination and taping (Figures 10.1 and 10.2). Second, certain anatomical variations such as arteria lusoria or subvlavian tortuosity/stenosis make the left radial approach more favorable. In fact, the incidence of right subclavian tortuosity has been reported to be 3 times as high compared to the left side.[2] In cases of severe tortuosity, catheter navigation may be more challenging, leading to prolonged procedure duration, increased radiation exposure,[3] and increased risk of vessel injury. In addition, avoiding the aortic arch in patients with severe atherosclerotic disease may prevent ischemic stroke due to embolus dislodgment from the arch.[1] Additional advantages of using the left radial side include the ease of forming

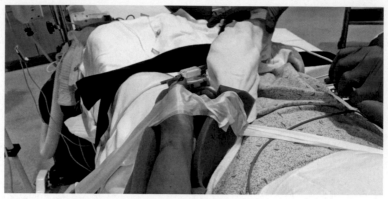

FIGURE 10.1 *Left hand positioned on top of the left groin.*

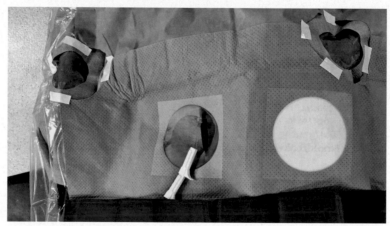

FIGURE 10.2 *Left wrist draped.*

the Simmons 2 catheter off the aortic valve to select the great vessels. This is because the wire selects the ascending aorta in contrast to the right radial access where the wire keeps directing down into the descending aorta. It is simpler to select the great vessels from the ascending aorta compared to the descending aorta (Figure 10.3). Also, selecting the left vertebral vessel is straightforward from the left side because the catheter does not require formation as opposed to the right-side approach.

After presenting the advantages of the left radial approach, it is important to know that one of the main limitations, which prevents the left side from being the primary approach, is the difficulty in selecting the left internal carotid artery, but there is no problem in selecting the left common carotid. This is due to an acute angle between the left subclavian artery and left common carotid artery. Such a limitation may be alleviated in the future by producing catheters specifically designed for the radial access.

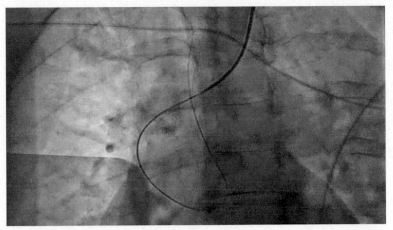

FIGURE 10.3 *Wire bouncing on the aortic valve while shaping the Simmons 2 catheter.*

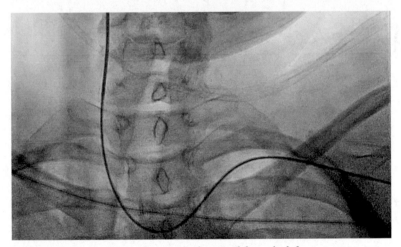

FIGURE 10.4 *Right internal carotid artery catheterized from the left.*

After anesthesia induction, the left wrist is positioned over the left groin to bring the access site closer to the operator standing on the right side. The left wrist is prepped and draped. The right wrist is positioned against the right hip of the patient in slight pronation and prepped and draped in the event that left radial access fails. Local lidocaine is administered in the left anatomic snuffbox, and the distal left radial artery is catheterized using ultrasound guidance via double-wall puncture and the Seldinger technique. If access at this site fails, the left radial artery is accessed at the wrist. Catheterization is achieved using a 5-French Prelude sheath. A mix of 2000 Units of heparin, 5 mg of nicardipine, and 200 μg of nitroglycerin is administered through the sheath. A radial run is then performed to evaluate the anatomy of the left radial artery. A 5 French Simmons 2 Penumbra catheter (Penumbra, Alameda, CA) is used to select the target vessels in its formed configuration in a similar fashion to right transradial angiography (Figures 10.4 and 10.5). After

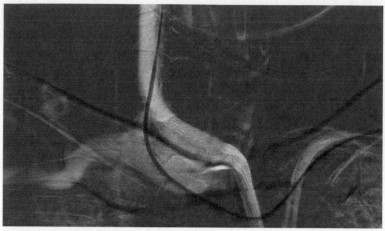

FIGURE 10.5 *Right vertebral artery catheterized from left.*

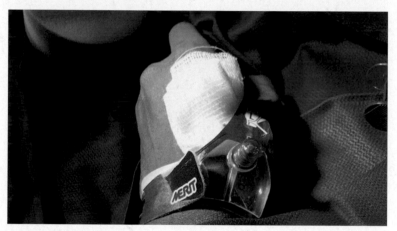

FIGURE 10.6 *Snuffbox band.*

the procedure is complete, the sheath is removed and a radial artery compression device is applied (Figure 10.6).

REFERENCES

1. Barros G, Bass DI, Osbun JW, et al. Left transradial access for cerebral angiography. *J Neurointerv Surg.* 2020;12(4):427–430.
2. Norgaz T, Gorgulu S, Dagdelen S. A randomized study comparing the effectiveness of right and left radial approach for coronary angiography. *Catheter Cardiovasc Interv.* 2012;80(2):260–264.
3. Sciahbasi A, Romagnoli E, Burzotta F, et al. Transradial approach (left vs right) and procedural times during percutaneous coronary procedures: TALENT study. *Am Heart J.* 2011;161(1):172–179.

Chapter 11

Use of Long Radial Sheaths for Radial Artery Spasm in Neurointerventions

EVAN LUTHER, PASCAL M. JABBOUR,
AND ERIC C. PETERSON

INTRODUCTION

Given the overwhelming data supporting transradial access (TRA) as a safer alternative to transfemoral access (TFA) in coronary interventions, neurointerventionalists have begun to transition away from femoral access. Recent studies in the neurointerventional literature have confirmed the safety benefits of TRA over TFA with significant decreases in access-site complications.[1-5] The key difference between TRA and TFA is the smaller size of the radial artery as compared to the femoral artery. This is advantageous in preventing access-site complications but also presents a new challenge because the smaller radial artery is prone to spasm. Large series have shown the incidence of radial artery spasm (RAS) to be as high as 50%, which can lead to unwanted crossovers to TFA.[6-9]

The new thin-walled radial artery vascular sheaths are designed with a thinner wall and smaller outer diameter than the conventional femoral sheaths to accommodate the smaller arterial diameter. However, the typical length of the radial artery sheath is approximately 10 cm, which is significantly shorter than the average radial artery length.

Vasospasm is only problematic when it is located in the radial artery because the caliber of the brachial artery is significantly larger than a guide catheter. Recently, long radial sheaths have been introduced that are designed to span the entire length of the radial artery, thereby preventing RAS from contacting the guide catheter. Herein, we describe our experience incorporating these long radial sheaths into our daily practice and describe the benefits associated with routine use of long radial sheaths as compared to the short radial sheaths.

LONG RADIAL SHEATH PLACEMENT PROTOCOL

The long radial sheath protocol was introduced at our institution in a stepwise fashion as a means to counteract RAS. Specifically, we evaluated all patients with a prior radial angiogram to determine if they had previously experienced RAS. If so, the long sheath was placed directly for their next transradial procedure. For those patients without a prior angiogram, we initially placed a short radial sheath. If RAS was encountered during arterial cannulation or seen on the radial angiogram, then we exchanged the short sheath for the long sheath. If RAS was not observed during access, then we continued with the procedure. However, if RAS was subsequently encountered during the procedure, we would again exchange for the long sheath. Figure 11.1 displays a flow diagram for our protocol.

STANDARD TRANSRADIAL ACCESS TECHNIQUES

Our technique for TRA has been described previously.[1,3,4,10–20] Briefly, the patient is placed supine on the angiography table and a pulse oximeter is placed on the ipsilateral thumb to monitor hand perfusion. A support board is placed inferior to the hand and lateral to the right knee, and padding is placed underneath the entire length of the arm terminating just distal to the fingertips so that the wrist remains level with the hip. For standard TRA, the hand is taped in a slightly supinated position to retract the thenar eminence, allowing access to the radial artery just proximal to the radial styloid. In distal TRA (dTRA), the hand is secured in a neutral position to expose the anatomic snuffbox.

Ultrasound is used in all cases without exception after prospective trial data demonstrated that it reduces procedure times.[21,22] Once appropriate backflow of blood through the sheath is identified, a radial artery angiogram is performed in all cases. Antispasmodic agents (usually 2.5 mg of verapamil and 200 µg of nitroglycerin) are given through the sheath in an effort to prevent RAS, and 65–70 units per kilogram of intravenous heparin is administered to protect against postprocedural radial artery occlusion.[1,4,11,12,14,16,18,23]

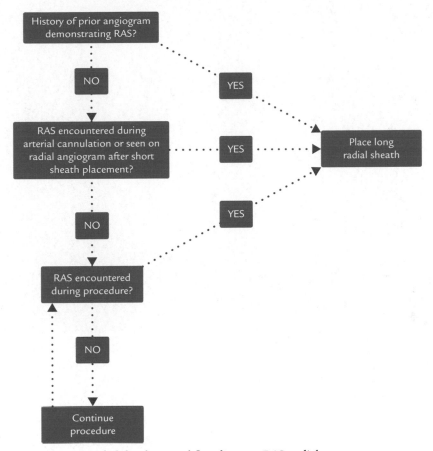

FIGURE 11.1 *Long radial sheath protocol flow diagram. RAS, radial artery spasm.*

LONG SHEATH EXCHANGE TECHNIQUE

Access and positioning are as described earlier. A short 10 cm 5, 6, or 7 French radial sheath (Terumo Glidesheath Slender) is placed and the radial angiogram is reviewed for spasm risk and radial anomalies. Specifically, the length and width of the exposed radial artery between its origin from the brachial artery and tip of the sheath are assessed. If clinical RAS is experienced during radial artery cannulation or significant radiographic RAS is seen on the angiogram, we proceed with exchanging for a long sheath. As with all radial artery angiograms, it is important to evaluate for radial artery anomalies such as a radial loop, a high-bifurcation radial origin, or radial tortuosity. Although unusual, they present unique technical challenges and may preclude the use of a long sheath. If a radial loop is present, microwire access to the brachial artery must be obtained and the loop straightened prior to placing the long sheath.

Once the decision has been made to exchange for a long sheath, a radial road map is obtained through the short sheath and a long 0.025 inch hydrophilic guide wire packaged

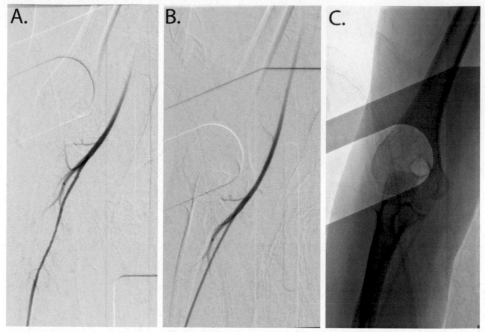

FIGURE 11.2 *Placement of a long radial sheath for radial artery spasm. (A) Radial angiogram demonstrating severe spasm. (B) Repeat radial angiogram after placement of a long sheath. (C) Native image confirming that the long sheath terminates at the brachial bifurcation.*

with the Merit 23 cm Ideal Sheath or Terumo 16 cm Glidesheath is navigated into the brachial artery. The long sheath is then exchanged over the wire for the short sheath with the introducer. The introducer and wire are then removed and back bled. A repeat radial artery angiogram is then performed to confirm placement of the sheath and to ensure that the radial artery no longer contains any segments of spasm. Figure 11.2 displays this. Systemic heparinization is then administered at this point.

We prefer the Merit Prelude Ideal 23 cm radial sheath (Merit Medical, South Jordan, UT) because the longer length consistently spans the entire length of the radial artery. The longest Glidesheath Slender is 16 cm (Terumo, Somerset, NJ) and often leaves a portion of the proximal radial artery uncovered and thus remains at risk of RAS. In particular, the 23 cm sheath is beneficial for covering the entire length of the radial artery for dTRA as the anatomic snuffbox is often 3–5 cm more distal than standard TRA.

ALTERNATIVE LONG SHEATH PLACEMENT TECHNIQUE

Rather than always exchanging for the long sheath, we place it during initial access for select cases when RAS is encountered during arterial cannulation or previous radial angiograms have demonstrated RAS. This has the advantage of faster procedure time, fewer steps, and less equipment used. This strategy is particularly useful for patients undergoing a TRA intervention that have had a prior TRA diagnostic angiogram. In these patients, the radial artery anatomy is known prior to puncture because we routinely obtain a radial artery angiogram as part of the diagnostic angiogram. If the radial artery is small or if spasm was encountered during the diagnostic angiogram, we routinely proceed directly with a long radial sheath for the intervention.

In cases where the patient does not have a prior radial angiogram, it is important to understand that there is a small chance that there is an underlying radial anomaly such as a radial loop or high-bifurcation radial origin. Unlike short sheaths, long sheaths often extend past radial loops, so it is important to be vigilant for the presence of a radial anomaly until a contrast injection is obtained to confirm correct placement into the brachial artery. There are two strategies for this. The first is to simply insonate the length of the radial artery with the ultrasound prior to puncture. The operator can thus confirm that the radial artery connects to the brachial artery at the level of the elbow and no radial loop or high radial takeoff exists.[24] The second strategy is to advance the microwire under fluoroscopy until it is past the elbow. Given the relative infrequency of radial anomalies (13.8%), if the wire goes smoothly, one can place the long radial sheath at this point. It is important to recognize that the wire can go smoothly even in the presence of a high-bifurcation radial origin or a radial artery loop. Contrast injection immediately following sheath placement is needed to confirm that the sheath is in the proximal radial or distal brachial artery prior to introducing the guide catheter.

If there is any question or concern with the appearance of the wire on fluoroscopy, the long sheath is advanced partially into the first 10 cm of the radial artery, the introducer is then removed, and the sheath is back bled. An angiogram is performed to confirm the radial artery anatomy. In the absence of any radial anomalies, the introducer is then replaced and the sheath is advanced completely over the microwire.

RATIONALE FOR USE OF LONG RADIAL SHEATHS

Although the use of the radial artery for endovascular procedures is associated with significantly lower complications as compared to the femoral artery, RAS can often preclude a transradial approach. Rates of RAS range between 6.8% and 50% in some large series. A systematic review evaluating 7197 patients undergoing TRA in coronary interventions reported an incidence of RAS of 14.7% and found that it did not differ based on the use of a 5F or 6F sheath.[7] Young age, female gender, small radial artery diameter, and unsuccessful first attempts at radial artery cannulation have all been identified as independent risk factors for the development of RAS.[7] In addition, anatomical variants such as high-bifurcation radial origins, radial loops, and radial tortuosity are also associated with increased risk of spasm.[25] Although trapped catheters are rare, even when the catheter is removed, the radial artery often remains significantly spasmed, precluding further radial access and necessitating conversion to femoral access.[11]

Previous studies have demonstrated that hydrophilic coating of sheaths and catheters significantly reduces RAS.[8,26–28] However with the use of a short radial sheath, the proximal portion of the radial artery is exposed and directly contacts a diagnostic or interventional catheter without hydrophilic coating. As the catheters are navigated into position in the great vessels, the radial artery endothelium experiences repetitive friction forces that lead to RAS. Figure 11.3(A,B) demonstrates this. While there are certainly radial arteries that are large enough to accommodate most systems, as catheter sizes increase, this scenario becomes increasingly relevant. Thus, even if the distal portion of a guide catheter has hydrophilic coating, it provides no benefit as that portion is quickly advanced into one of the great vessels, leaving the uncoated proximal portion of the catheter in contact with the exposed radial artery.

The use of a long radial sheath obviates all of this by providing a stable hydrophilic conduit from the skin to the brachial artery, at which point the large diameter of the brachial artery renders spasm a nonissue (Figure 11.3C). Thus, the radial artery never comes into contact with the dynamic guide catheter. Many patients have a sufficiently large radial artery (>2 mm) to allow a case to be performed with a short sheath without event. However, in our experience RAS can occur even when the radial artery diameter appeared large enough to have a low risk of spasm and was seen even with 5F systems. As such, we have developed a very low threshold for use of these long sheaths in our practice. Specifically, we have found three clinical scenarios where use of a long sheath is particularly helpful.

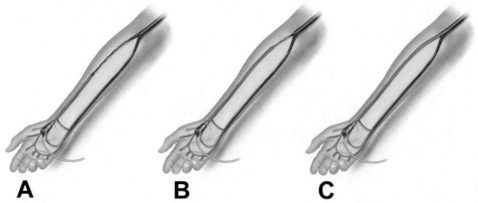

A   **B**   **C**

FIGURE 11.3 *Radial sheath lengths in patients with radial artery spasm. (A) 10 cm short sheath leaves a significant portion of the proximal radial artery exposed. (B) 16 cm long sheaths often still leave a small portion of the proximal radial artery exposed. (C) 23 cm long sheaths consistently span the entire length of the radial artery.*

CLINICAL SCENARIOS WHERE LONG SHEATH IS HELPFUL: DIAGNOSTIC ANGIOGRAMS

As we have moved the majority of our diagnostic practice to dTRA, we have utilized the 5F 23 cm Merit Ideal sheath with increasing frequency. The snuffbox puncture site is 3–5 cm more distal than traditional TRA, which means that, once placed, the sheath will terminate more distally, leaving more exposed endothelium in the proximal radial artery for spasm to occur. For patients with a large-caliber radial artery on ultrasound, we will often still begin with a short radial sheath but convert to the long sheath if the radial artery is small or spasm is encountered during cannulation. In addition, if we placed a short sheath and the radial angiogram reveals a small radial artery or severe spasm distal to the sheath, we immediately exchange for a long sheath.

Left radial access for neurointerventions is significantly less common than in interventional cardiology. Nonetheless, for many left vertebral interventions the preferred access site is the left radial artery. As we have described, the preferred approach to the left radial artery is via the snuffbox approach with the arm bent and positioned over the patients abdomen.[10,29] While this allows for a significantly more ergonomic set-up for the operator, the distal puncture site again leads to more exposed radial artery at the end of a short sheath. A long radial sheath directly addresses this issue.

CLINICAL SCENARIOS WHERE LONG SHEATH IS HELPFUL: RADIAL ARTERY ANOMALIES

Radial anomalies are also an indication for a long sheath in our practice. Radial loops and high-bifurcation radial origins have higher risk of RAS because both anomalies result in increased radial artery surface area exposed to diagnostic catheters without hydrophilic coating.[25] Figure 11.4 displays a radial loop and a high-bifurcation radial origin, respectively. As such, both are ideal cases for placement of long radial sheaths. If a radial loop is present, wire access to the brachial artery must be obtained and the loop straightened prior to placing the long sheath.

CLINICAL SCENARIOS WHERE LONG SHEATH IS HELPFUL: INTERVENTIONS

The rationale and anatomy described earlier applies for interventions as well. Short sheaths suffice as long as the radial artery distal to the sheath is of sufficient caliber to accommodate an interventional catheter without development of RAS. We now use 6F Prelude Ideal 23 cm sheaths (Merit, South Jordan, UT) in all our 6F interventions if prior

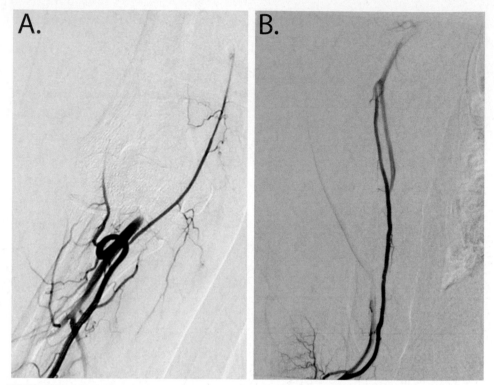

FIGURE 11.4 *Radial anomalies. (A) Radial loop. (B) High-bifurcation radial origin.*

radial angiograms demonstrated any RAS in order to reduce the risk of crossover. This has become even more relevant as we have begun to use dTRA for interventions as well.

We have also found an increasingly larger role for the long 7F 23 cm radial sheaths. Prospective data have found rates of radial artery occlusion (RAO) for these 7F sheaths to be very low (<5%), and placement of them allows for a radial arterial line to be provided to anesthesia during our procedure, further reducing patient punctures and procedure times.[30] This is particularly helpful during procedures requiring bilateral radial access, such as complex posterior circulation aneurysms or balloon test occlusions, in which anesthesia does not have access to a radial artery for invasive blood pressure monitoring.[10]

SHEATH CHOICE

There are currently two thin-walled radial sheaths available: the Glidesheath Slender (Terumo, Somerset, NJ) and the Ideal sheath (Merit, South Jordan, UT), and both exist in 5F, 6F, and 7F sizes. The Terumo slender sheaths (Terumo, Somerset, NJ) are available in 10 or 16 cm lengths, and the Merit radial sheaths are available in 7, 11, or 23 cm lengths (Merit, South Jordan, UT). While we prefer the hydrophilic coating of the

Terumo Glidesheath Slender, only the 23 cm sheath consistently covers the entire length of the radial artery (Figure 11.1C). Thus, at present our preferred radial sheath is the Glidesheath Slender for short sheath cases and the 23 cm Merit Ideal sheath for long sheath cases. As always, we rely heavily on the radial artery angiogram to make decisions regarding sheath choice and length.

CONCLUSIONS

RAS remains one of the most common complications associated with TRA in neuro-endovascular procedures. The use of long 23 cm hydrophlic radial sheaths may prevent RAS because they protect the full length of the radial artery and diminish the repetitive friction forces of the catheter against the radial artery. We have found that implementation of a long sheath protocol to address RAS significantly reduced rates of access-site conversions due to clinical RAS in diagnostic cerebral angiography and neurointerventional procedures performed via TRA. Given the impressive results on lowering crossover rates, we now use this protocol for all TRA procedures performed at our institution.

ACKNOWLEDGMENTS

Roberto Suazo for designing the figures displayed in this manuscript.

REFERENCES

1. Chen SH, Snelling BM, Sur S, Shah SS, McCarthy DJ, Luther E, et al. Transradial versus transfemoral access for anterior circulation mechanical thrombectomy: comparison of technical and clinical outcomes. *J Neurointerv Surg.* 2019;11(9):874–878.
2. Li Y CS, Spiotta AM, Jabbour P, Levitt MR, Kan P, et al. Lower complication rates associated with transradial versus transfemoral flow diverting stent placement. *J Neurointerv Surg.* 2020;12(2):22–29.
3. McCarthy DJ, Chen SH, Brunet MC, Shah S, Peterson E, Starke RM. Distal radial artery access in the anatomical snuffbox for neurointerventions: case report. *World Neurosurg.* 2019;122:355–359.
4. Snelling BM, Sur S, Shah SS, Caplan J, Khandelwal P, Yavagal DR, et al. Transradial approach for complex anterior and posterior circulation interventions: technical nuances and feasibility of using current devices. *Oper Neurosurg (Hagerstown).* 2019;17(3):293–302.
5. Sweid A, Starke RM, Herial N, Chalouhi N, Xu V, Shivashankar K, et al. Transradial approach for the treatment of brain aneurysms using flow diversion: feasibility, safety, and outcomes. *J Neurosurg Sci.* 2019;63(5):509–517.
6. Coghill EM, Johnson T, Morris RE, Megson IL, Leslie SJ. Radial artery access site complications during cardiac procedures, clinical implications and potential solutions: The role of nitric oxide. *World J Cardiol.* 2020;12(1):26–34.
7. Kristic I, Lukenda J. Radial artery spasm during transradial coronary procedures. *J Invasive Cardiol.* 2011;23(12):527–531.

8. Rathore S, Stables RH, Pauriah M, Hakeem A, Mills JD, Palmer ND, et al. Impact of length and hydro-philic coating of the introducer sheath on radial artery spasm during transradial coronary intervention: a randomized study. *JACC Cardiovasc Interv.* 2010;3(5):475–483.

9. Kim SH, Kim EJ, Cheon WS, Kim MK, Park WJ, Cho GY, et al. Comparative study of nicorandil and a spasmolytic cocktail in preventing radial artery spasm during transradial coronary angiography. *Int J Cardiol.* 2007;120(3):325–330.

10. Luther E, McCarthy D, Silva M, Nada A, Strickland A, Chen S, et al. Bilateral transradial access for complex posterior circulation interventions. *World Neurosurg.* 2020;139:101–105.

11. Brunet MC, Chen SH, Peterson EC. Transradial access for neurointerventions: management of access challenges and complications. *J Neurointerv Surg.* 2019;17(8):120–126.

12. Brunet MC, Chen SH, Sur S, McCarthy DJ, Snelling B, Yavagal DR, et al. Distal transradial access in the anatomical snuffbox for diagnostic cerebral angiography. *J Neurointerv Surg.* 2019;11(7):710–713.

13. Chen SH, Brunet MC, Sur S, Yavagal DR, Starke RM, Peterson EC. Feasibility of repeat transradial access for neuroendovascular procedures. *J Neurointerv Surg.* 2019;122(3):119–125.

14. Chen SH, McCarthy DJ, Sheinberg D, Hanel R, Sur S, Jabbour P, et al. Pipeline embolization device for the treatment of intracranial pseudoaneurysms. *World Neurosurg.* 2019;127:e86–e93.

15. Chen SH, Peterson EC. Pearls and pitfalls: radial first for neurointervention. *Endovascular Today.* 2019. Available from evtoday.com/articles/2019-nov/pearls-and-pitfalls-radial-first-for-neurointervention.

16. Chen SH, Snelling BM, Shah SS, Sur S, Brunet MC, Starke RM, et al. Transradial approach for flow diversion treatment of cerebral aneurysms: a multicenter study. *J Neurointerv Surg.* 2019;11(8):796–800.

17. Shah SS, Snelling BM, Brunet MC, Sur S, McCarthy DJ, Stein A, et al. Transradial mechanical thrombectomy for proximal middle cerebral artery occlusion in a first trimester pregnancy: case report and literature review. *World Neurosurg.* 2018;120:415–419.

18. Snelling BM, Sur S, Shah SS, Khandelwal P, Caplan J, Haniff R, et al. Transradial cerebral angiography: techniques and outcomes. *J Neurointerv Surg.* 2018;10(9):874–881.

19. Snelling BM, Sur S, Shah SS, Marlow MM, Cohen MG, Peterson EC. Transradial access: lessons learned from cardiology. *J Neurointerv Surg.* 2018;10(5):487–92.

20. Sur S, Snelling B, Khandelwal P, Caplan JM, Peterson EC, Starke RM, et al. Transradial approach for mechanical thrombectomy in anterior circulation large-vessel occlusion. *Neurosurg Focus.* 2017;42(4):E13.

21. Bernat I, Abdelaal E, Plourde G, Bataille Y, Cech J, Pesek J, et al. Early and late outcomes after primary percutaneous coronary intervention by radial or femoral approach in patients presenting in acute ST-elevation myocardial infarction and cardiogenic shock. *Am Heart J.* 2013;165(3):338–343.

22. Seto AH, Roberts JS, Abu-Fadel MS, Czak SJ, Latif F, Jain SP, et al. Real-time ultrasound guidance facilitates transradial access: RAUST (Radial Artery access with Ultrasound Trial). *JACC Cardiovasc Interv.* 2015;8(2):283–291.

23. Spaulding C, Lefevre T, Funck F, Thebault B, Chauveau M, Ben Hamda K, et al. Left radial approach for coronary angiography: results of a prospective study. *Cathet Cardiovasc Diagn.* 1996;39(4):365–370.

24. Lo TS, Nolan J, Fountzopoulos E, Behan M, Butler R, Hetherington SL, et al. Radial artery anomaly and its influence on transradial coronary procedural outcome. *Heart.* 2009;95(5):410–415.

25. Ruiz-Salmeron RJ, Mora R, Masotti M, Betriu A. Assessment of the efficacy of phentolamine to prevent radial artery spasm during cardiac catheterization procedures: a randomized study comparing phentolamine vs. verapamil. *Catheter Cardiovasc Interv.* 2005;66(2):192–198.

26. Caussin C, Gharbi M, Durier C, Ghostine S, Pesenti-Rossi D, Rahal S, et al. Reduction in spasm with a long hydrophylic transradial sheath. *Catheter Cardiovasc Interv.* 2010;76(5):668–672.

27. Kiemeneij F, Fraser D, Slagboom T, Laarman G, van der Wieken R. Hydrophilic coating aids radial sheath withdrawal and reduces patient discomfort following transradial coronary intervention: a randomized double-blind comparison of coated and uncoated sheaths. *Catheter Cardiovasc Interv.* 2003;59(2):161–164.

28. Koga S, Ikeda S, Futagawa K, Sonoda K, Yoshitake T, Miyahara Y, et al. The use of a hydrophilic-coated catheter during transradial cardiac catheterization is associated with a low incidence of radial artery spasm. *Int J Cardiol.* 2004;96(2):255–258.

29. Barros G, Bass DI, Osbun JW, Chen SH, Brunet MC, Peterson EC, et al. Left transradial access for cerebral angiography. *J Neurointerv Surg.* 2020;12(4):427–430.

30. Aminian A, Iglesias JF, Van Mieghem C, Zuffi A, Ferrara A, Manih R, et al. First prospective multicenter experience with the 7 French Glidesheath slender for complex transradial coronary interventions. *Catheter Cardiovasc Interv.* 2017;89(6):1014–1020.

CHAPTER 12

Closure Techniques

KALYAN SAJJA, ERIC C. PETERSON, AND
PASCAL M. JABBOUR

THE SUPERFICIAL LOCATION, SMALL SIZE, AND EASE WITH WHICH THE radial artery can be compressed eliminate the need for the types of closure devices that are used for femoral arteriotomy closure.[1] Mechanical compression for radial artery access closure can be considered superior to manual approach as it exerts a stable and continuous pressure on the artery.[1] Radial artery occlusion (RAO) is one of the few complications closely associated with radial artery access-site closure, and a good closure technique aims to minimize the incidence of RAO.

TECHNIQUE FOR MANUAL COMPRESSION

The introducer sheath is pulled out by a few centimeters, and pressure with three fingers is applied over the puncture site. The sheath is pulled out completely until some bleeding is visible, which is thought to purge the prothrombotic material and also serves as an indicator for radial artery antegrade flow.[1] Manual pressure is maintained for about 10 minutes or longer as needed for hemostasis. Longer compression times are needed with the use of larger sheaths or the use of antiplatelets, anticoagulants, or fibrinolytics.

Many different variations of inexpensive compression devices are available. These can be strapped onto the patient's wrist to apply compression at the arterial puncture site. The older generation devices were static compression devices and were not suitable for gentle compression or patent hemostasis techniques. The newer devices come with an inflatable pressure bladder and a transparent structure to observe the access site. The simplest of these devices are cheaper and easier to use. The more commonly used compression bands are Vasc band Hemostat (Teleflex, PA), TR band (TR Band; Terumo, Somerset, NJ), and PreludeSYNC Distal hemostasis device (Merit Medical Inc., UT). Vascular compression devices improve patient comfort and allow the operator, nursing staff, and the catheterization laboratory to move forward quickly. They can be especially helpful when prolonged compression is needed.

TECHNIQUE FOR APPLYING A COMPRESSION DEVICE

Apply Betadine on the insertion site and dry it prior to applying the compression device. The introducer sheath is retracted by a few centimeters and the compression device is strapped to the wrist. The marker of the compression band's balloon is positioned just proximal to the puncture site and the balloon is inflated. About 10 cc of air is adequate for the majority of the patients.[2] We typically use about 7 cc for most of our patients. The sheath is then removed while making sure there is no bleeding. Hemostatic pressure in the compression band is slowly deflated. If pulsatile oozing of the blood is noted, then the deflation is stopped and 1 cc of air is injected back into the balloon. This simple and uncomplicated technique ensures that hemostasis is achieved with a gentle compression. The compression device is left inflated for about 30 minutes. If the patient is on anti-platelets or anticoagulants, the compression device is left inflated for up to 1 hour before hemostatic pressure weaning protocol is started in the postoperative unit. After the stipulated time, the compression device is gradually deflated by 1–2 cc every 5–10 minutes until final hemostasis. If pulsatile bleeding is noted at any point, 1 cc of air is injected back in, and the weaning protocol is paused for a few minutes before proceeding. After hemostasis is achieved, dressing with a tegaderm bandage is applied. Motor and sensory function and perfusion distal to the access site are checked regularly after hemostasis (see Figure 12.1).

Longer compression and pressure weaning times might be needed for larger introducer sheath sizes, when anticoagulation cannot be interrupted, or in patients who get fibrinolytics for stroke. There is no clear consensus on the optimal hemostatic pressure weaning protocol. In the CRASOC I, II, and III studies (Compression of Radial Arteries Without Occlusion), shorter compression times resulted in lower rates of RAO.[3] If the patient has an unfavorable plethysmogram, SpO_2 drop, or symptoms

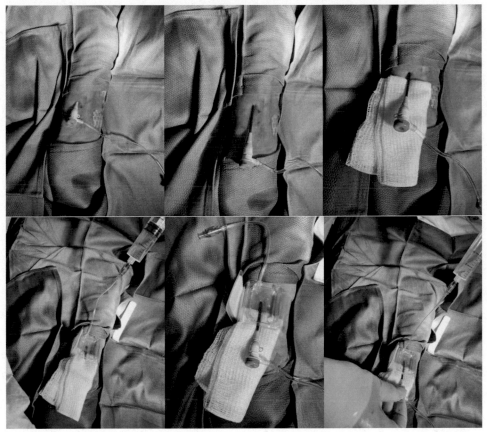

FIGURE 12.1 *Steps in the application of a Vasc Band Hemostat for the closure of radial access site.*

from low perfusion, the compression device is removed and manual compression is selectively applied on the radial artery. This ensures perfusion from the ulnar artery while the radial artery is occluded. Assessment for forearm or wrist hematoma is important at every stage because compartment syndrome can occur if the hematoma is not promptly identified and managed. Compression for a slightly longer time usually reduces the hematoma.

Pancholy et al. described the patent hemostasis technique that is defined as maintenance of antegrade flow in the radial artery during hemostatic compression.[4] Following the placement of the compression device with a gentle compression technique, the ulnar artery is compressed manually while the pulse wave is monitored on the pulse oximeter ("reverse Barbeau test"). If anterograde flow in the radial artery is absent as noted on the plethysmography, the pressure of the radial artery compression is decreased in an attempt to re-establish anterograde radial artery flow without sacrificing hemostasis (patent hemostasis). Once radial artery patency is confirmed with a persistent waveform in the presence of a compressed ulnar artery, the patient is transitioned to the recovery area. It is hypothesized that an increase in radial artery flow due to ulnar flow interruption leads to flow-mediated vasodilation of the radial artery. This then ameliorates any residual spasm and lowers the risk of RAO. If radial artery patency and antegrade flow on plethysmography is not confirmed, compression of the ulnar artery can be continued while maintaining patent hemostasis with the band and pulse oximeter in place, and this sequence is usually effective at re-establishing patency.[5] This technique has been shown to significantly lower the incidence of RAO by adjusting the compression to a "just needed" intensity for obtaining hemostasis and by maintaining radial patency during compression.

Another technique that can be concomitantly used to reduce the incidence of RAO is prophylactic ulnar artery compression. A second compression device is placed on the ulnar artery and is maximally inflated. This is hypothesized to increase the peak blood flow into the radial artery, leading to improved rates of radial recanalization by promoting localized fibrinolysis.[6] In the PROPHET-II study, 30-day RAO was significantly reduced in patients with patent hemostasis and prophylactic ulnar compression compared with standard patent hemostasis alone (0.9% vs. 3.0%; $p = 0.0001$).[7]

Complicated techniques, including the patent hemostasis technique and techniques using mean arterial pressure (RACOMAP study[8]) to ensure radial artery patency, have had limited operational adoption in catheterization laboratories around the world.[8,9] This has been driven by the need for larger involvement of the postprocedural care team with repeated evaluations of radial antegrade flow, making a rather simplistic and inexpensive process of hemostatic compression a significantly more complex process.[8]

The technique for the distal radial arteriotomy closure (a.k.a. anatomical snuffbox) is similar to the technique for the standard radial access closure as described earlier. It typically takes significantly less pressure for the compression device in the distal radial access closure compared to the standard radial access. Merrit's PreludeSync Distal hemostasis device (a.k.a. snuffbox band) is designed for the distal radial access compression and provides comfortable compression for patients. This device has better opposition and compression at the distal radial site compared to other compression bands which are designed for compression at the standard radial access site and comes in two configurations for use with the right and left distal radial access closure. Vasc band also works reasonably well for compression of the distal radial access site. In our experience, the Terumo TR band might not work very well for the closure of the distal radial access site. If that is the only device available, then using a larger (rather than the regular size) Terumo band might save face (see Figure 12.2).

We do not use hemostatic bandages routinely. A selected group of patients, who receive fibrinolytic agents and anticoagulants, might benefit from the use of hemostatic bandages in combination with compression devices.[10] Some of the examples of the numerous hemostatic bandages are QuikClot Interventional hemostatic bandage, Clo-Sur PAD (Scion Cardiovascular, Miami, FL), Chito-Seal (Abbott Vascular, Redwood City,

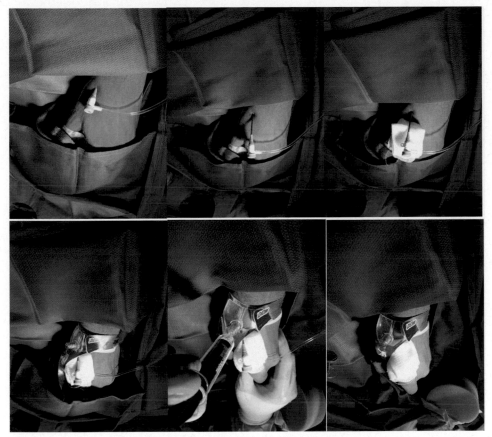

FIGURE 12.2 *Steps in the application of PreludeSYNC distal hemostasis device for closure of a distal radial access site.*

CA), and Neptune Pad (Biotronik, Berlin, Germany). These pads are coated with procoagulant material to enhance coagulation and hemostasis. They also selectively absorb water molecules and concentrate the coagulation factors, resulting in faster time to hemostasis. The Kaolin-based procoagulant pads can activate XII factor and accelerate the coagulation cascade,[11] while the Chitosan-based procoagulant pads use positively charged chitosan molecules to attract the negatively charged blood cells and platelets, thus promoting blood clotting.[10] The Clo-Sur P.A.D. works outside of the clotting cascade.[12] The compression time required for hemostasis is reduced when these hemostasis pads are used concomitantly with compression bands.[10,11] This translates to a reduced incidence of RAO.[7] Any additional cost, however, has to be taken into consideration when hemostatic pads are used. A disadvantage when used alone is that the titrability feature that is required for patent hemostasis is not available.

RAO can be an infrequent and asymptomatic complication of radial artery catheterization in most of the cases. Absence of radial pulse after TRA procedures may be a strong indicator of RAO. However, a palpable pulse does not exclude the diagnosis of RAO:

collateral blood flow, mainly through the anterior interosseous artery, can supply the periphery of the radial artery distally to the occlusion and give a false impression of radial artery patency. Thus, the incidence of RAO varies based on palpation versus using a more objective method such as an ultrasound. RAO can often go undiagnosed, and its true incidence is likely underestimated. Since RAO is asymptomatic most of the time, the true incidence of RAO in clinical practice is considered to be even higher. Spontaneous recanalization of the radial access approaches 50% after 30 days. RAO persisted after 30 days in 3.3%–5.5% of the patients.[13,14,15] This factor also contributes to systematic underestimation when assessment of radial patency is not performed based on the absence of symptoms or based on the presence of palpable pulse. Patency is better evaluated with clinical testing as the reverse Barbeau's test and with Doppler ultrasonography.[16] Early studies reported higher incidence of RAO in up to 33% or higher proportion of the cases.[17] More recently, the pooled incidence rate of early RAO was found to be between 5% and 7.7%.[13]

The clinical significance of RAO remains controversial as RAO is asymptomatic most of the time. Sometimes it can be subclinical, giving symptoms only in cold weather or during exertion.[14] Rarely, cases of hand ischemia due to RAO have been described.[18]

Late spontaneous recanalization occurs in a significant fraction of the patients within 30–90 days after procedure.[19,20] Despite this, RAO must be minimized as it is one of the most common reasons for failure of future use of this safe route.[12]

The primary pathophysiologic mechanism underlying RAO appears to be thrombosis, with contributions from endothelial injury, inflammation, intimal or medial dissection, and vasospasm.[21] Imaging studies have demonstrated localized vascular trauma, intimal thickening, and vessel narrowing upon reaccess.[21] Sluggish flow at the access site and trauma to the artery that occurs either during the access or by denuding the endothelium during sheath placement lead to a prothrombotic state and ensue in RAO (see Boxes 12.1 and 12.2).[12,21]

Excessive compression after sheath removal is a strong predictor of RAO.[22,25] In the CRASOC I trial, 13 cc air was used for compression, which led to 9% rate of RAO. This fell to 2% in CRASOC II and III trials, where 10 cc was used and reduced compression time (1.5 hours) was used.[3] The 10 cc used for the CRASOC II and III studies achieved hemostasis for 89% of patients and adding 2 cc resulted in hemostasis for 97% of TRA.[3] Every 1 hour increase in duration after 1.5 hours resulted in a 49% increase in RAO and 14% increase in RAO for every 1 cc of air pushed in after 10 cc.[3]

The PROPHET II study randomized 3000 patients to the patent hemostasis technique with the TR Band device versus patent hemostasis and simultaneous compression of the ulnar artery.[7] The patent hemostasis group had a 4.3% RAO at 24 hours versus 1% for the group with added ulnar artery compression. The inflatable TR Band has less incidence of RAO when compared to other noninflatable hemostatic devices.[7,14,31] In another

---

BOX 12.1
FACTORS THAT PROMOTE RADIAL ARTERY OCCLUSION

Age
Sex
Body weight
Height
Serum creatinine
Peripheral artery disease
Number of punctures
DM
Absence of antegrade flow when obtaining hemostasis
Smoking

Sources: [3,16,19,20,22]

BOX 12.2
FACTORS THAT REDUCE RADIAL ARTERY OCCLUSION

Gentle compression technique
Smaller size of the access
Duration of compression
"Patent hemostasis" technique
Immediate postprocedural sheath removal
Dose-dependent use of heparin
Use of distal transradial access
Use of longer sheaths
Postprocedural/prehemostasis intra-arterial nitroglycerin
Postprocedural treatment with ASA or coumadin
Smaller sheath-to-artery ratio

Sources: [6,22,23,24,25,26,27,28,29,30]

---

study, using inflatable TR Band compression device compared to a noninflatable band reduced the risk of RAO at 24 hours (4.4% vs. 11.2%, $p < 0.005$) and at 30 days (3.2% vs. 7.2%, $p < 0.05$) after the procedure.[32]

Once RAO is suspected based on the absence of a previously palpable radial pulse, then confirmation should be obtained with either plethysmography or radial artery duplex ultrasonography. If RAO is noted, then ipsilateral ulnar artery compression for 1 hour can recanalize a significant number of patients.[6] Otherwise, conservative medical management with anticoagulation for 4 weeks usually results in recanalization in a significant number of cases (87%; Zankl et al.).[33] Most RAO cases do not mandate definitive therapy beyond reassurance, observation, and rarely analgesia in the event of forearm discomfort. Rhyne and Mann described a successful use of coronary angioplasty techniques to restore patency of a recently occluded radial artery with complete resolution of the presenting symptoms of hand ischemia.[18] However, insufficient data exist for the routine use of invasive strategies. Transient ulnar artery compression might be a noninvasive and simple method to restore radial artery patency in the immediate postoperative setting. Bernat et al. evaluated the role of transient compression of the ipsilateral ulnar artery for 1 hour to promote radial artery recanalization. In their study, ulnar artery compression was performed for 1 hour by maximally inflating TR Band for patients with evidence of RAO on ultrasound. With the combination of heparin and ulnar artery compression, incidence of RAO was reduced from 2.9% to 0.8% $(p = 0.03)$.[6]

Some practitioners perform an angiogram prior to closure and if there is angiographic evidence of vasospasm, radial cocktail/vasodilators can be administered through the sheath. This is thought to decrease subjective discomfort which some patients complain about afterward. A nitrate patch sometimes can be used postoperatively in severe vasospasms. A prospective randomized study demonstrated that 500 µg of intra-arterial nitroglycerin delivered through the sheath at the conclusion of the procedure was associated with a significant decrease in RAO assessed via ultrasound at 1 day post procedure compared to placebo.[34]

A good closure technique of radial access site translates to a lower incidence of RAO and other such complications which prevent future access to this safe site.

REFERENCES

1. Petroglou D, Didagelos M, Chalikias G, Ziakas D, Tsigkas G, Hahalis G, Koutouzis M, Ntatsios A, Tsiafoutis I, Hamilos M, Kouparanis A, Konstantinidis N, Sofidis G, Pancholy SM, Karvounis H, Bertrand OF, Ziakas A. Manual versus mechanical compression of the radial artery after transradial coronary Angiography. *J Am Coll Cardiol Intv.* 2018;11(11):1050–1058.

2. Koutouzis M, Maniotis C, Avdikos G. Prevention of radial artery occlusion after transradial catheterization. *J Am Coll Cardiol Interv.* 2017;10(1):103.

3. Dangoisse V et al. Usefulness of a gentle and short hemostasis using the transradial band device after transradial access for percutaneous coronary angiography and interventions to reduce the radial artery occlusion rate (from the prospective and randomized CRASOC I, II, and III studies. *Am J Cardiol,* 2017;120(3):374–379.

4. Pancholy S, Coppola J, Patel T, Roke-Thomas M. Prevention of radial artery occlusion—Patent hemostasis evaluation trial (PROPHET study): A randomized comparison of traditional versus patency documented hemostasis after transradial catheterization. *Cathet Cardiovasc Intervent.* 2008;72:335–340. doi:10.1002/ccd.21639

5. Edris A et al. Facilitated patent haemostasis after transradial catheterisation to reduce radial artery occlusion. *EuroIntervention*. 2015;11(7):765–771. doi:10.4244/EIJV11I7A153

6. Bernat I et al. Efficacy and safety of transient ulnar artery compression to recanalize acute radial artery occlusion after transradial catheterization *Am J Cardiol*. 2008;107(11):1698–1701.

7. Pancholy SB, Bernat I, Bertrand OF, Patel TM. Prevention of radial artery occlusion after transradial catheterization: the PROPHET-II randomized trial. *JACC: Cardiovasc Interv*. 2016;9(19):1992–1999. https://doi.org/10.1016/j.jcin.2016.07.020.

8. Bertrand OF, Rao SV, Pancholy S, Jolly SS, Rodés-Cabau J, Larose E, Costerousse O, Hamon M, Mann T. Transradial approach for coronary angiography and interventions: results of the first International Transradial Practice Survey. *JACC: Cardiovasc Interv*. 2010;3(10):1022–1031. https://doi.org/10.1016/j.jcin.2010.07.013.

9. Cubero JM, Lombardo J, Pedrosa C, et al. Radial compression guided by mean artery pressure versus standard compression with a pneumatic device (RACOMAP). *Cathet Cardiovasc Interv*. 2009;73:467–472.

10. Kang S-H et al. Hemostasis pad combined with compression device after transradial coronary procedures: A randomized controlled trial. *PloS One* 2017;12(7):e0181099. doi:10.1371/journal.pone.0181099

11. Politi L, Aprile A, Paganelli C, Amato A, Zoccali GB, Sgurfa F, Monopoli D, Rossi R, Modena MG, Sangiori GM. Randomized clinical trial on short-time compression with kaolin-filled pad: a new strategy to avoid early bleeding and subacute radial artery occlusion after percutaneous coronary intervention. *J Interv Cardiol*. 2011;24:65–72. doi:10.1111/j.1540-8183.2010.00584

12. Shroff A, Siddiqui S, Burg A, Singla I. Identification and management of complications of transradial procedures. *Curr Cardiol Rep*. 2013;15(4):1–9.

13. Rashid M et al. Radial artery occlusion after transradial interventions: a systematic review and meta-analysis. *J Am Heart Assoc*. 2016;5(1):e002686. doi:10.1161/JAHA.115.002686

14. Zwaan EM, Koopman AG, Holtzer CA, et al. Revealing the impact of local access-site complications and upper extremity dysfunction post transradial percutaneous coronary procedures. *Neth Heart J*. 2015;23(11):514–524. doi:10.1007/s12471-015-0747-9

15. Sinha SK, Jha MJ, Mishra V, Thakur R, Goel A, Kumar A, Singh AK, Sachan M, Varma CM, Krishna V. Radial artery occlusion-incidence, predictors and long-term outcome after transradial catheterization: Clinico-Doppler ultrasound-based study (RAIL-TRAC study). *Acta Cardiol*. 2017;72:318–327. doi:10.1080/00015385.2017.1305158

16. Avdikos G et al. Radial artery occlusion after transradial coronary catheterization. *Cardiovasc Diag Ther*. 2017;7(3):305–316. doi:10.21037/cdt.2017.03.14

17. Lefevre T, Thebault B, Spaulding C, Funck F, Chaveau M, Guillard N, Chalet Y, Bellorini M, Guerin F. Radial artery patency after percutaneous left radial artery approach for coronary angiography: the role of heparin. *Eur Heart J*. 1995;16:293–297.

18. Rhyne D, Mann T. Hand ischemia resulting from a transradial intervention: Successful management with radial artery angioplasty. *Cathet Cardiovasc Intervent*. 2010;76:383–386.

19. Agostoni P, Biondi-Zoccai GG, de Benedictis ML, et al. Radial versus femoral approach for percutaneous coronary diagnostic and interventional procedures; Systematic overview and meta-analysis of randomized trials. *J Am Coll Cardiol*. 2004;44(2):349–356. doi:10.1016/j.jacc.2004.04.034

20. Barbosa RA, Andrade MVA, Andrade PB, Rinaldi FS, Bienert IRC, Nogueira EF, Tebet MA, Esteves VC, Mattos LAP, Labrunie A. Use of a selective radial compression device to prevent radial artery occlusion after coronary invasive procedure. *Revista Brasileira de Cardiologia Invasiva* 2014;22(2):115–119. https://dx.doi.org/10.1590/0104-1843000000020

21. Kotowycz MA, Dzavík V. Radial artery patency after transradial catheterization. *Circ Cardiovasc Interv*. 2012;5(1):127–133. doi:10.1161/CIRCINTERVENTIONS.111.965871

22. Costa F, van Leeuwen MA, Daemen J, et al. The Rotterdam Radial Access Research: Ultrasound-Based Radial Artery Evaluation for Diagnostic and Therapeutic Coronary Procedures. *Circ Cardiovasc Interv*. 2016;9(2):e003129. doi:10.1161/CIRCINTERVENTIONS.115.003129

23. Dangoisse V, Guédès A, Chenu P, et al. Usefulness of a Gentle and Short Hemostasis Using the Transradial Band Device after Transradial Access for Percutaneous Coronary Angiography and Interventions to Reduce the Radial Artery Occlusion Rate (from the Prospective and Randomized CRASOC I, II, and III Studies). *Am J Cardiol.* 2017;120(3):374–379. doi:10.1016/j.amjcard.2017.04.037

24. Pancholy SB, Patel TM. Effect of duration of hemostatic compression on radial artery occlusion after transradial access. *Cathet Cardiovasc Intervent.* 2012;79:78–81. doi:10.1002/ccd.22963

25. Wagener JF, Rao SV. Radial artery occlusion after transradial approach to cardiac catheterization. *Curr Atheroscler Rep.* 2015;17(3):489. doi:10.1007/s11883-015-0489-6

26. Takeshita S et al. Comparison of frequency of radial artery occlusion after 4Fr versus 6Fr transradial coronary intervention (from the Novel Angioplasty USIng Coronary Accessor Trial). *Am. J. Cardiol.* 2014;113(12):1986–1989.

27. Takeshita S, Tanaka S, Saito S. Coronary intervention with 4-French catheters. *Cathet. Cardiovasc. Intervent.* 2010;75:735–739. doi:10.1002/ccd.22308

28. Lotan C et al. Transradial approach for coronary angiography and angioplasty. *Am J Cardiol.* 1995;76(3):164–167.

29. Bernat I et al. Efficacy and safety of transient ulnar artery compression to recanalize acute radial artery occlusion after transradial catheterization. *Am J Cardiol.* 2011;107(11):1698–1701.

30. Koutouzis MJ, Maniotis CD, Avdikos G, Tsoumeleas A, Andreou C, Kyriakides ZS. Ulnar artery transient compression facilitating radial artery patent hemostasis (ULTRA): a novel technique to reduce radial artery occlusion after transradial coronary catheterization. *J Inv Cardiol.* 2016;28:451–454.

31. Rathore S, Stables RH, Pauriah M, Hakeem A, Mills JD, Palmer ND, Perry RA, Morris JL. A randomized comparison of TR band and radistop hemostatic compression devices after transradial coronary intervention. *Cathet Cardiovasc Intervent.* 2010;76:660–667. doi:10.1002/ccd.22615

32. Pancholy SB. Impact of two different hemostatic devices on radial artery outcomes after transradial catheterization. *J Inv Cardiol.* 2009;21:101–104.

33. Zankl AR, Andrassy M, Volz C, et al. Radial artery thrombosis following transradial coronary angiography: incidence and rationale for treatment of symptomatic patients with low-molecular-weight heparins. *Clin Res Cardiol.* 2010;99:841–847.

34. Dharma S, Kedev S, Patel T, et al. A novel approach to reduce radial artery occlusion after transradial catheterization: postprocedural/pre hemostasis intra-arterial nitroglycerin. *Cathet Cardiovasc Interv.* 2015;85:818–825.

CHAPTER 13

Pediatric Transradial Approach

KARIM HAFAZALLA, FADI AL SAIEGH,
ERIC C. PETERSON, AND PASCAL M. JABBOUR

INTRODUCTION

Neuroendovascular approaches have quickly become a mainstay approach for treat-ment of several neurological pathologies. Whether it be embolization of vascular malformations, mechanical thrombectomy for an ischemic stroke, or serving as an adjunct to open surgery, neuroendovascular surgery has revolutionized the way pa-tient care is provided. Traditionally, these procedures were achieved via transfemoral access. With large-caliber vessels for access and a relatively straightforward trajectory to the cerebral vasculature, this access point was a natural first choice as endovascular approaches were being introduced to neurosurgical practice. As the field continued to progress, the radial artery was introduced as an alternative access site. The RIVAL trial was a landmark study for this movement, showing radial access had equal efficacy of percutaneous coronary intervention while having a safer complication profile when compared to femoral access.[1] While transradial access became the primary approach for cardiovascular procedures in the past decade, it has only recently gained traction in neurosurgical circles. As more centers adopt this new approach, it has become clear that transradial access is an extremely valuable access site for neuroendovascular surgery. Its advantages include lower risk for complications, which can be fatal using the transfemoral route, higher patient satisfaction, and shorter hospital stays.[2,3] Those advantages are not unique to the adult population but are, in fact, even more pronounced in pediatrics. With a much smaller total blood volume, a retroperitoneal hematoma can be deadly in pediatric patients. In addition, keeping patients on flat bed rest for hemostasis at the groin is much more challenging in young children and often requires continuous intravenous sedation.[4]

Transradial Access for Diagnostic Cerebral Angiography

Transradial access has had well-established success in coronary angiographies of both adults and children, and as far back as the early 2000s, some centers have published data on this approach for cerebral angiographies.[5-9] Gradually, as supportive evidence has continued to grow for the transradial route, some interventional providers have transitioned their practice to a "radial first" approach. Promising results from high-volume centers showed that transradial approach angiograms were safe and effective, with a successful angiographic catheterization of preplanned vessels cited between 88% and 97%.[10-12]

Zussman and colleagues published the first prospective study assessing transradial access for cerebral angiographies.[10] They acknowledged their 88% success rate, while still high, showed the relative inexperience their providers had with this access as compared to the transfemoral alternative and was an indication of what neurointerventionalists at large should expect when first trialing this access. Their highest cause of failure was gaining access to the radial artery (6% of cases). Peripheral vascular disease, unfamiliar anatomy, vasospasm, and the radial artery's small size can make successful cannulation of the radial artery tenuous.

While more challenging in pediatrics, the advantages are quite substantial. They include early mobilization of patients since flat bed rest is not required as it is with transfemoral puncture for hemostasis at the groin. This also obviates the need for continuous intravenous dexmedetomidine or other sedatives, which is fraught with its own risks. Furthermore, transradial approaches eliminate one of the most feared complications of femoral punctures in the pediatric population, such as acute limb ischemia or hematoma, which can be life threatening because of the small intravascular volume in this population. In an early report by Srinivasan et al., the authors report their experience with 37 diagnostic angiograms. The average radial artery diameter cannulated was 2.09 mm.[13] Despite these challenges, complications with access quickly become minimal with further experience. An interventional cardiology study cited their failure of cannulation went down from 10% to 1% over time.[14]

TECHNICAL DETAILS OF RADIAL ARTERY
CATHETERIZATION IN PEDIATRICS

Typically, the patient's right wrist is for radial artery catheterization. The wrist is positioned in slight supination and extension, which brings the radial artery closer to the skin surface. The subcutaneous is carefully injected with local lidocaine, and ultrasound is used to visualize the radial artery and catheterize it. A MicroPuncture kit 4Fr introducer sheath is most commonly used in the senior author's practice (Figure 13.1). Once blood return is obtained, a "radial cocktail" of 500 Units of heparin, 1 mg of nicardipine, and 50 µg of nitroglycerin are administered intra-arterially. This cocktail reduces the risk of spasm and thrombus formation. Based on the procedure planned, a guide catheter may or may not be necessary. For example, for a targeted angiogram of the right internal circulation, a guide catheter may not be needed (Figures 13.2 and 13.3). However, any catheterization of the left carotid circulation will require a 4Fr Simmons 2 guide catheter because it is nearly impossible to cross to the left side with only a microcatheter. In Our practice 3 YO is the youngest we would go transradial. Once the procedure is concluded, the sheath is removed and a transradial inflatable band is used to hold pressure over the puncture site for "patent hemostasis" for about 2 hours (Figure 13.4). During this time, oxygenation of the hand is continuously monitored using pulse oximetry.

Transradial Access for Neurointerventions

Transradial access has begun to change the treatment of pediatric populations. Majmundar and colleagues were the first to publish results on this matter, highlighting a case series of four patients requiring embolization.[15] Conditions treated included nasopharyngeal angiofibroma, right internal carotid artery pseudoaneurysm, and arteriovenous

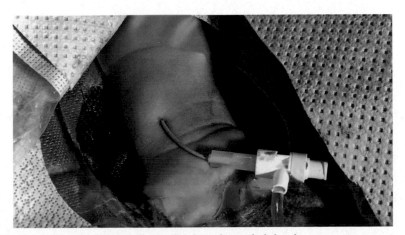

FIGURE 13.1 *The introducer of the 4Fr sheath used as radial sheath.*

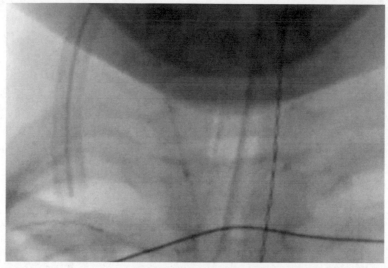

FIGURE 13.2 *Microcatheter in a case of intra-arterial chemotherapy for retinoblastoma.*

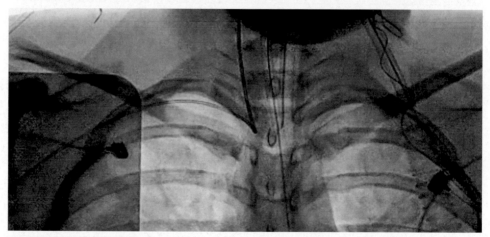

FIGURE 13.3 *A 4Fr Simmons 2 catheter in a case of intra-arterial chemotherapy.*

malformation. Only one patient had vasospasm, and no conversion to transfemoral access was required. These findings were further supported by Srinivasan and colleagues, who reported vasospasm in only eight pediatric patients and switching to femoral access in five cases out of their 61 procedures.[13]

Another facet of pediatric neurointerventional care that transradial access has begun to impact is in the administration of intra-arterial chemotherapy (IAC).[4] In a series of five patients, Al Saiegh and colleagues showed safe and efficacious administration of IAC for retinoblastoma without complication and all patients went home the same day.[4] Furthermore, IAC for retinoblastoma typically requires multiple sequential treatments. A study by Chen and colleagues involving 104 patients showed the radial artery could be safely used for up to six procedures with minimal complications (5.3% of cases), further

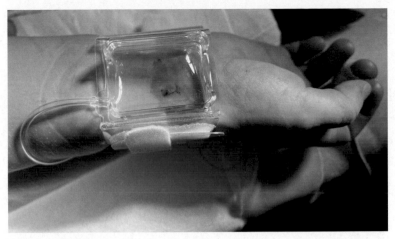

FIGURE 13.4 *A radial band in place.*

supporting the case for transradial access in IAC administration.[16] As IAC is now considered a first-line treatment for retinoblastoma, these studies show substantial promise for the future of this treatment modality.[17–19]

Advantages of Transradial over Transfemoral Access for Neurointerventions in Pediatrics

Utilizing the radial artery comes with a host of advantages when compared to the femoral artery. In the preoperative setting, patients who are anticoagulated are less worrisome if receiving a transradial procedure, as the risk of clinically significant hematoma is much less than with the femoral artery.[9,12] From the operator's perspective, its location in the wrist means a simpler set-up in the operating room. The ability to abduct the arm away from the body allows for more room for the operator, and the patient's body habitus has less of an impact on patient set-up.[20] While unfamiliar anatomy in the transradial route can be a concern for neurointerventionalists, the learning curve is swift—Snelling and colleagues showed a decrease in mean fluoroscopy time per vessel as their neurointerventionalists gained more experience.[11] In fact, they claimed that only 15 angiograms were needed for improved efficiency with no corresponding increase in patient complications.

With regards to complications, radial access shows superiority in many aspects relative to femoral access.[21] Retroperitoneal hematomas are a feared complication of transfemoral access, potentially resulting in circulatory failure. This is especially true in the pediatric population, where only a small amount of blood loss could lead to exsanguination.[4,21] With radial access, hematomas are rare and typically clinically nonsignificant. Another benefit of transradial access is its distal position in the upper extremity. Combined with collateral circulation from the ulnar artery, it results in an exceedingly low-risk radial artery occlusion (as low as 1%) and limb ischemia.[11,15] Even when they do occur, they are usually clinically silent.[15] Given the femoral artery's more proximal location in the leg, loss of limb is a much more significant risk.

Patients similarly prefer the convenience of the transradial access over the transfemoral alternative. Due to its superficial location in the wrist, postoperative pain, immobilization times, and hospital stays overall are all less compared to transfemoral access procedures.[3,4,15] Snelling and colleagues were able to quantify their patients' satisfaction, with 86.2% of patients reporting "none" to "mild" wrist discomfort postoperatively. And of those that had had a prior procedure via transfemoral access, 67% responded they would prefer the transradial access.[11] Khanna et al. had even more convincing findings, with only 6% of responders preferring the transfemoral approach.[3] From a pediatric perspective, reduction in postoperative immobilization time is a substantial benefit. Transfemoral access in pediatric populations typically requires manual pressure, as pediatric femoral arteries are typically too small for arterial closure devices.[13] This combination of manual pressure requirement and prolonged immobilization period often results in a sedation requirement for infants and young children to comply. The transradial access reduces this necessity, allowing for pediatric populations to mobilize more quickly, use fewer medications, and utilize arterial closure devices.

CONCLUSIONS

It is clear that transradial access has many benefits in the neuroendovascular field. While it is still relatively slow to be adopted, continuous data have emerged to support its ability to be used in a variety of procedures while conferring minimal complication risks. The pediatric population stands to benefit even more so, as the radial access affords the ability to perform multiple procedures using the radial artery, reduced sedation requirements, and low risk of hematoma upon gaining access. While the transfemoral route may be more comfortable for some providers currently, the transradial route can be adopted relatively quickly and provides several benefits for both patient and operator. It has revolutionized the field of interventional cardiology, and as more centers adopt a "radial first" methodology, so too will neurosurgical practices.

REFERENCES

1. Jolly SS, Yusuf S, Cairns J, et al. Radial versus femoral access for coronary angiography and intervention in patients with acute coronary syndromes (RIVAL): a randomised, parallel group, multicentre trial. *Lancet.* 2011;377(9775):1409–1420.
2. Khanna O, Mouchtouris N, Sweid A, et al. Transradial approach for acute stroke intervention: technical procedure and clinical outcomes. *Stroke Vasc Neurol.* 2020;5(1):103–106.

3. Khanna O, Sweid A, Mouchtouris N, et al. Radial artery catheterization for neuroendovascular procedures. *Stroke.* 2019;50(9):2587–2590.

4. Al Saiegh F, Chalouhi N, Sweid A, et al. Intra-arterial chemotherapy for retinoblastoma via the transradial route: technique, feasibility, and case series. *Clin Neurol Neurosurg.* 2020;194:105824. doi:10.1016/j.clineuro.2020.105824

5. Agostoni P, Biondi-Zoccai GG, de Benedictis ML, et al. Radial versus femoral approach for percutaneous coronary diagnostic and interventional procedures; systematic overview and meta-analysis of randomized trials. *J Am Coll Cardiol.* 2004;44(2):349–356.

6. Irving C, Zaman A, Kirk R. Transradial coronary angiography in children and adolescents. *Pediatr Cardiol.* 2009;30(8):1089–1093.

7. Lee DH, Ahn JH, Jeong SS, Eo KS, Park MS. Routine transradial access for conventional cerebral angiography: a single operator's experience of its feasibility and safety. *Br J Radiol.* 2004;77(922):831–838.

8. Matsumoto Y, Hongo K, Toriyama T, Nagashima H, Kobayashi S. Transradial approach for diagnostic selective cerebral angiography: results of a consecutive series of 166 cases. *Am J Neuroradiol.* 2001;22(4):704–708.

9. Nohara AM, Kallmes DF. Transradial cerebral angiography: technique and outcomes. *Am J Neuroradiol.* 2003;24(6):1247–1250.

10. Zussman BM, Tonetti DA, Stone J, et al. A prospective study of the transradial approach for diagnostic cerebral arteriography. *J Neurointerv Surg.* 2019;11(10):1045–1049.

11. Snelling BM, Sur S, Shah SS, et al. Transradial cerebral angiography: techniques and outcomes. *J Neurointerv Surg.* 2018;10(9):874–881.

12. Sattur MG, Almallouhi E, Lena JR, Spiotta AM. Illustrated Guide to the Transradial Approach for Neuroendovascular Surgery: A Step-by-Step Description Gleaned From Over 500 Cases at an Early Adopter Single Center. *Oper Neurosurg (Hagerstown).* 2020;19(2):181–189. doi:10.1093/ons/opaa153

13. Srinivasan VM, Hadley CC, Prablek M, et al. Feasibility and safety of transradial access for pediatric neurointerventions. *J Neurointerv Surg.* 2020;12(9):893–896. doi:10.1136/neurintsurg-2020-015835

14. Ball WT, Sharieff W, Jolly SS, et al. Characterization of operator learning curve for transradial coronary interventions. *Circ Cardiovasc Interv.* 2011;4(4):336–341.

15. Majmundar N, Patel P, Dodson V, et al. First case series of the transradial approach for neurointerventional procedures in pediatric patients [published online ahead of print, 2020 Jan 31]. *J Neurosurg Pediatr.* 2020:1–5. doi:10.3171/2019.12.PEDS19448

16. Chen SH, Brunet MC, Sur S, Yavagal DR, Starke RM, Peterson EC. Feasibility of repeat transradial access for neuroendovascular procedures. *J Neurointerv Surg.* 2020;12(4):431–434.

17. Dalvin LA, Kumari M, Essuman VA, et al. Primary intra-arterial chemotherapy for retinoblastoma in the intravitreal chemotherapy era: five years of experience. *Ocul Oncol Pathol.* 2019;5(2):139–146.

18. Sweid A, Hammoud B, Weinberg JH, et al. Intra-arterial chemotherapy for retinoblastoma in infants ≤10 kg: 74 treated eyes with 222 IAC sessions. *AJNR Am J Neuroradiol.* 2020;41(7):1286–1292. doi:10.3174/ajnr.A6590.

19. Rojanaporn D, Chanthanaphak E, Boonyaopas R, Sujirakul T, Hongeng S, Ayudhaya SSN. Intra-arterial chemotherapy for retinoblastoma: 8-year experience from a tertiary referral institute in Thailand. *Asia Pac J Ophthalmol (Phila).* 2019;8(3):211–217.

20. Catapano JS, Fredrickson VL, Fujii T, et al. Complications of femoral versus radial access in neuroendovascular procedures with propensity adjustment. *J Neurointerv Surg.* 2020;12(6):611–615.

21. Joshi KC, Beer-Furlan A, Crowley RW, Chen M, Munich SA. Transradial approach for neurointerventions: a systematic review of the literature. *J Neurointerv Surg.* 2020;12(9):886–892. doi:10.1136/neurintsurg-2019-015764

CHAPTER 14

Intraoperative Transradial Angiogram

AHMAD SWEID, ERIC C. PETERSON, AND
PASCAL M. JABBOUR

INTRAOPERATIVE ANGIOGRAM (IOA) IS A VALUABLE TOOL FOR CEREBRO-vascular surgery. IOA allows early diagnosis and identification of any residue and obviates the need for postoperative diagnostic angiogram. It confirms surgical outcomes for a variety of pathologies such as aneurysm occlusion and parent vessel patency, arteriovenous malformation resection, dural fistula ligation, bypass patency, and adequate carotid revascularization after endarterectomy.[1] Though there are alternatives, such as indocyanine green fluorescence (ICGA) angiography, formal angiography remains the gold standard because it overcomes the limitations of ICGA. Femoral access has been the main approach for IOA with an excellent safety profile.[2] Recently the radial approach has been gaining wide interest among neurointerventionalists, and there are several advantages for the radial approach over the femoral approach in IOA.[3]

Access to the radial artery is technically easier than the femoral artery, especially in obese patients with a large pannus. Also, surgical positions such as lateral prone and three-quarters prone make IOA using a femoral approach more challenging.[3] The ergonomics of the C-arm are superior using the radial approach (Figure 14.1). The arm position on a radiolucent arm board allows clear visualization of the catheter and guide wire

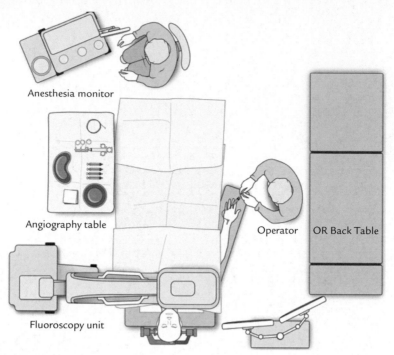

FIGURE 14.1 *Schematic view of the disposition of the transradial approach intraoperative angiogram. OR, operating room.*

from the access point into the subclavian artery during live fluoroscopy. Such positioning eliminates the need to follow the catheter through the femoral and iliac vessels into the descending aorta and arch, which is often limited by several objects such as the nonradiolucent operating table pedestal, Mayfield head holder attachment, and cardiac monitoring wires. Also, in tall patients it may be more challenging to obtain a groin run because the fluoroscopy unit is blocked by the base of the operating table. The radial angiogram is quick to complete, in less than 10 minutes, which gives enough time to avoid any ischemic complications in the event a parent vessel is compromised. At the completion of the procedure, hemostasis is much easier using the radial approach by simply placing a vascular band, which is less painful compared to femoral closure devices and allows early mobilization. The latter is very important because it avoids keeping the patient flat for 4–6 hours and permits raising the head of the bed if need be. Also, it avoids delaying extubation, as it is not uncommon for the anesthesiologist to keep the patient intubated to keep him or her flat to avoid the risk of aspiration. Additionally, if the patient inadvertently moves the leg or coughs during anesthesia emergence, it would not increase the risk of bleeding from the femoral access site. One major challenge that one has to be aware of is that image acquisition of the aortic arch is challenging during IOA in certain positions other than supine, while in prone positions angiographic views are obtained by inverting the image on the C-arm. Also, catheter navigation is challenging in patients in the three-quarters prone position.

After induction of general anesthesia, the right wrist is positioned and taped against the hip of the patient in slight pronation and extension to bring the radial artery to the surface. The right wrist and bilateral groins are sterilized and draped in a standard sterile fashion. The distal radial artery at the anatomic snuffbox is accessed; alternatively, the radial artery at the wrist is used. Access is obtained in supine position before the final position for the craniotomy. Craniotomy is subsequently performed to access the lesion. After treatment of the lesion, IOA studies are acquired under a portable single-plane fluoroscopy unit. The operator stands at the patient's right side while the fluoroscopy unit and angiography table are at the patient's left side, which allows for a comfortable working space. The fluoroscopy monitor faces the operator. A radial artery angiogram is initially performed through the sheath, and a 5 French Simmons 2 Penumbra catheter (Penumbra, Alameda, CA) is then navigated over an 0.035 inch soft Glidewire (Terumo Medical Corporation, Somerset, NJ) into the subclavian artery under anteroposterior fluoroscopy and using road map guidance. If possible, the Glidewire is advanced directly to the right or left common carotid artery depending on the vessel of interest. The procedure is performed as earlier described. Angiograms are reviewed by the operating neurosurgeon, and intraoperative adjustments are performed and angiography is repeated as needed until the goals of surgery are achieved. At the conclusion of the cerebral angiogram, all catheters and wires are removed. Once the craniotomy is closed, the arterial sheath is removed and a TR Band is placed (Terumo Medical Corporation). The compression band is inflated with air and slowly, sequentially deflated after 1 hour. The PrecludeSync distal band (Merit Medical, South Jordan, UT) is used for sheaths placed in the anatomic snuffbox.

REFERENCES

1. Tang G, Cawley CM, Dion JE, Barrow DL. Intraoperative angiography during aneurysm surgery: a prospective evaluation of efficacy. *J Neurosurg.* 2002;96(6):993–999.
2. Osbun JW, Patel B, Levitt MR, et al. Transradial intraoperative cerebral angiography: a multicenter case series and technical report. *J Neurointerv Surg.* 2020;12(2):170–175.
3. Chalouhi N, Sweid A, Al Saiegh F, et al. Initial experience with transradial intraoperative angiography in aneurysm clipping: technique, feasibility, and case series. *World Neurosurg.* 2020;134:e554–e558.

CHAPTER 15

Access-Site Complications of the Transfemoral Approach

STEPHANIE H. CHEN, PASCAL M. JABBOUR, AND ERIC C. PETERSON

INTRODUCTION

The femoral artery has been the most commonly used access site for endovascular procedures. However, complications via the femoral approach can lead to significant morbidity and even mortality. Complications range from mild bruising and discomfort to life-threatening retroperitoneal hematomas. Other complications include femoral artery dissections, pseudoaneurysms, occlusions, fistulas, and femoral nerve injuries. In this chapter, we review the rate of femoral access-site complications as well as strategies for treatment.

ANATOMY AND TECHNIQUE

The best strategy for mitigating femoral access-site complications is avoidance with the use of appropriate cannulation technique. The external iliac artery arises from the common iliac artery and crosses under the inguinal ligament to become the common femoral artery. The common femoral artery resides in the femoral triangle, which is bordered by the inguinal ligament superiorly, sartorius laterally, and adductor longus medially. The femoral artery should be cannulated at the base of the femoral triangle, above the bifur-cation of the femoral artery. The goal is to cannulate the femoral artery where the artery overlies the middle third of the femoral ahead so that it can be compressed against the femoral head to achieve hemostasis. Fluoroscopy as well as palpation of maximal femoral pulsation can be used to locate the artery in relation to the femoral head. Additionally, routine ultrasound use has been shown to decrease access-site complications, time to ac-cess, and accidental venipunctures in femoral arterial access.[1]

HEMATOMA

Access-site hemorrhages are common complications of interventional procedures using the transfemoral approach. Risk factors for developing a groin hematoma include obesity, use of anticoagulation, insufficient manual compression, large sheaths, early ambulation, and peripheral vascular disease.[2] In a systematic review of randomized neuroendovascu-lar clinical trials, groin hemorrhage rates ranged from 0.23% to 10.68% with an average of 2.89%.[2] Differences in occurrence rates are partly due to differences in defining what constitutes a hematoma with variable size thresholds. However, the rates in the neuroen-dovascular trial are consistent with the rates of groin hematomas reported in cardiology studies as well. Yatskar et al. found that a hematoma is the most frequent periprocedural complication and occurs in 2% to 12% of percutaneous coronary intervention cases.[3]

RETROPERITONEAL HEMATOMAS

Retroperitoneal hematomas are a rare but potentially life-threatening complication of femoral puncture. They can occur due to a femoral puncture above the level of the in-guinal ligament or from an uncontrolled expanding groin hematoma. It can be difficult to diagnose due to the nonspecific symptoms of suprainguinal tenderness and fullness, back or lower abdominal pain, and lower extremity pain. Left untreated, the patient could be-come quickly hemodynamically unstable; thus, treatment involves intensive care unit ob-servation, blood transfusion, fluid resuscitation, and reversal of anticoagulation. Patients may require surgical intervention by intra-arterial embolization, balloon tamponade, or open surgery if conservative measures fail.

PERIPHERAL ARTERY OCCLUSIONS

Unlike the transradial approach, peripheral artery occlusion after a transfemoral approach is a severe complication that can lead to lower extremity ischemia and loss of the limb.

Arterial occlusions may occur due to thrombosis, stenosis, or dissection. Three neuro-endovascular randomized controlled trials reported incidence rates between 0.23% and 2.04% with an average rate of 0.5%.[4,5,6] Higher incidence rates ranging from 0.14% and 6.86% were associated with the use of arterial closure devices.[7,8] Signs and symptoms include lower limb pain, claudication, cold limb, pallor, parasthesias, and pulselessness. Diagnosis can be made with a duplex ultrasound, and aggressive endovascular or surgical treatment should be pursued. Blood flow can be restored by balloon angioplasty, thromboectomy or thrombolysis, stents, or open surgical thrombectomy and repair.

FEMORAL ARTERY DISSECTIONS AND PSEUDO-ANEURYSMS

Femoral artery dissections are a disruption of the layers of the wall of the artery. They are usually caused by the needle or guide wire entering into the wall of the vessel during arterial puncture. Dissections typically do not require treatment and remain asymptomatic as anterograde blood flow holds the flap down. However, dissections resulting in complete occlusion of the femoral artery require treatment to prevent limb ischemia.

A femoral pseudoaneurysm is a full thickness arterial wall injury with an associated hematoma. The incidence rate of a femoral artery pseudoaneurysm ranges between 0.23% and 3.23% after a transfemoral approach in the neuronendovascular literature.[2] Small pseudoaneurysms less than 3 cm can be observed, and they tend to resolve spontaneously within 1 month. Treatment strategies include prolonged compression, percutaneous thrombin injections into the pseudoaneurysm, as well as coil embolization, stents, and open surgical repair.

ARTERIOVENOUS FISTULAS

Arteriovenous (AV) fistulas are a rare complication of femoral artery catheterization wherein an abnormal communication between the artery and the vein occur. The main risk factor is puncture below the femoral bifurcation at the superficial femoral artery; however, other risk factors include hypertension, female gender, left groin puncture, and anticoagulation.[2] AV fistulas can be conservatively observed if small and not hemodynamically significant. However, if the patient becomes symptomatic with increased swelling and tenderness, increased shunting leading to limb claudication or high-output heart failure, treatment should be pursued. Treatment options include prolonged bandaging, percutaneous stenting or coil embolization, or open surgical repair.

ARTERIAL CLOSURE DEVICES

There are a variety of arterial closure devices. The two main types of active devices are collagen plug devices (i.e., AngioSeal, Terumo) and suture mediated closure devices (Perclose, Abbott Vascular). Passive closure devices enhance manual compression with the assistance of mechanical clamps (FemStop, Abbott Vascular) or external patches and plugs (Mynx, Cordis and Vascade, Cardiva). The literature comparing the use of arterial closure devices to manual compression is variable. A prospective multicenter trial by Sato et al. showed significantly fewer groin hematomas associated with Angioseal as compared to manual compression (5.04% vs 34.55%, $p < 0.001$) as well as shorter hemostasis time (4.4 vs. 150.7 minutes, $p < 0.001$).[9] However, other meta-analyses have shown similar rates of vascular complications when comparing closure devices and mechanical compression.[2,10]

OTHER COMPLICATIONS

Other rare complications that have been reported are infections and neurologic complications. Infections complications include local abscess, cellulitis, or sepsis, and the most common organisms are *Staphylococcus aureas* and *Staphylococcus epidermidis*. Incidence ranges from 0.23% to 2.15%. Sterile techniques are recommended for all catheterization procedures; however, the routine use of prophylactic antibiotics is not recommended.[11] Neurologic complications include femoral neuropathy, parasthesias, and chronic pain. Femoral neuropathy is most commonly seen in association with a large hematoma or pseudoaneurysm creating compression of the femoral nerve. Retroperitoneal hematomas that cause pressure on the femoral nerve may result in permanent weakness of the upper leg and leg pain. Pressure on the femoral cutaneous nerve can also result in a sensory neuropathy.

REFERENCES

1. Seto AH et al. Real-time ultrasound guidance facilitates femoral arterial access and reduces vascular complications: FAUST (Femoral Arterial Access With Ultrasound Trial). *JACC Cardiovasc Interv.* 2010;3(7):751–758.
2. Oneissi M et al. Access-site complications in transfemoral neuroendovascular procedures: a systematic review of incidence rates and management strategies. *Oper Neurosurg (Hagerstown).* 2020;20(7):32–140.
3. Yatskar L et al. Access site hematoma requiring blood transfusion predicts mortality in patients undergoing percutaneous coronary intervention: data from the National Heart, Lung, and Blood Institute Dynamic Registry. *Cathet Cardiovasc Interv.* 2007;69(7):961–966.
4. Broderick JP et al. Endovascular therapy after intravenous t-PA versus t-PA alone for stroke. *N Engl J Med.* 2013;368(10):893–903.

5. Saver JL et al. Solitaire flow restoration device versus the Merci Retriever in patients with acute ischaemic stroke (SWIFT): a randomised, parallel-group, non-inferiority trial. *Lancet.* 2012;380(9849):1241–1249.

6. Sakai N et al. Efficacy and safety of REVIVE SE thrombectomy device for acute ischemic stroke: River JAPAN (Reperfuse Ischemic Vessels with Endovascular Recanalization Device in Japan). *Neurol Med Chir (Tokyo).* 2018;58(4):164–172.

7. Gandhi CD et al. Neuroendovascular management of emergent large vessel occlusion: update on the technical aspects and standards of practice by the Standards and Guidelines Committee of the Society of NeuroInterventional Surgery. *J Neurointerv Surg.* 2018;10(3):315–320.

8. Geyik S et al. The safety and efficacy of the Angio-Seal closure device in diagnostic and interventional neuroangiography setting: a single-center experience with 1,443 closures. *Neuroradiology.* 2007;49(9):739–746.

9. Sato M et al. Usefulness of an access-site hemostasis device in neuroendovascular treatment. *Acta Neurochir (Wien).* 2017;159(12):2331–2335.

10. Nikolsky E et al. Vascular complications associated with arteriotomy closure devices in patients undergoing percutaneous coronary procedures: a meta-analysis. *J Am Coll Cardiol.* 2004;44(6):1200–1209.

11. Sohail MR et al. Infectious complications of percutaneous vascular closure devices. *Mayo Clin Proc.* 2005;80(8):1011–1015.

CHAPTER 16

How to Start Your Radial Practice

EVAN LUTHER AND ERIC C. PETERSON

CONVERTING TO THE TRANSRADIAL APPROACH (TRA) AS THE DEFAULT method for performing neurointervention in your practice is likely to be one of the more rewarding changes you can make. It should be viewed as a minimally invasive neurointervention, and all of the benefits of minimally invasive techniques across the surgical spectrum can be expected here as well. The patient feedback, nursing feedback, and technical stimulation of TRA are large drivers of this. Pascal and I have spent considerable time trying to convey our best advice for how to actually perform neurointervention via TRA. However, like all techniques, there is a learning curve. Similar to many changes in practice that involve more than just doing the procedure differently, understanding the different stakeholders can make a big difference in your journey. What follows is my advice for how to set up your radial practice for success.

PRINCIPLE 1: COMMIT TO 50 CONSECUTIVE CASES

One of the biggest errors when converting to TRA is to dabble. It takes time to learn the puncture. It takes time to learn the table set-up. It takes time to learn how to form the sim and manage arch variants. It takes time for your techs to learn the set-up. It takes time for your nurses to understand that their patients no longer need to lay flat for hours. Once you are past that hump, then it is smooth sailing. The cases are easy, patients are happy, and the machine hums along. However, there is some effort that is needed to get there. You will be slow. You will make mistakes. Your techs will complain. Your nurses will not understand. If you get discouraged and stop after a few cases, you will never fix all these issues and will just go back to the groin. This is a great disservice to your patients.

The good news is that most people follow the same adoption process (Figure 16.1). There is some initial interest and a few cases are done. There is some initial complaining and frustration, but then the patients start saying, "That was so much better than the leg. I want that every time." Nurses start saying, "Wow, doc, ever since you started this radial stuff the patients are so much happier. They are sitting up in the ICU in a chair texting their kids rather than lying flat complaining of back pain." You start getting faster and more consistent. It becomes fun. Pretty soon groin access seems barbaric. But it takes a push to get there.

If you dabble, then you will never get over the hump. It does not matter if it is 50 diagnostics or interventions. However you do it, get to 50. Many users get there well before 50. However, you have to be confident that this is better for your patients and commit to the work to get there.

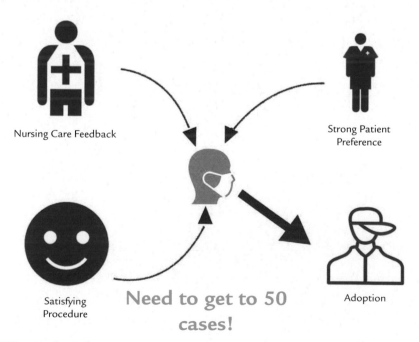

Nursing Care Feedback

Strong Patient Preference

Satisfying Procedure

Need to get to 50 cases!

Adoption

FIGURE 16.1 *Radial conversion process.*

PRINCIPLE 2: ENGAGE WITH YOUR TECHS AND NURSES FROM THE START

Unless your techs cross cover interventional cardiology where they do TRA routinely, then they are going to resist changing to TRA. That isn't because it is slower or harder. It is actually just as fast if not faster to prep than transfemoral. It's just that humans don't like to change behaviors. So rather than force it, engage them. Tell them up front: "There is a safer way to gain access, and it's much better for patients. We are going to start doing cases via radial access, and I need your help. It will take a little bit to learn, but we have to keep doing it until we get over the learning curve. Going forward, I would prep both radial and femoral for every case." Same story with the nurses. They especially get very engaged with anything that is better for their patients. Tell them the plan, as well as how the postoperative care will be different.

Once you engage the techs and nurses, see Principle 1—do not dabble! Consistency is a force multiplier here. If everyone knows that the patients should be set up for radial access *every single time*, then there is minimal complaining. It is simply how things are done. However, if you dabble and they don't really know if you are doing this or not, you will face continued resistance throughout your journey. You are the captain. You have to lead as a consistent and confident example.

With regard to nursing, we have found that structured postprocedure order sets are essential to streamlining the transition. Many hospital systems are appropriately protocol driven, so simply telling the RN that "this patient doesn't need any femoral precautions" often results in patients spending even more time in bed since there is confusion as to what the exact orders are. A simple template of our order set is shown in Figure 16.2.

PRINCIPLE 3: YOU DON'T HAVE TO START WITH JUST DIAGNOSTICS

Many people think you should start slow with diagnostics and then go into progressively more challenging interventions. This is reasonable, and it is how I learned. However, that was because no one seemed to be doing it at that time and I didn't have anyone to show me the details. That is no longer the case. There have been countless articles, talks, and webinars (now even a book!) on this topic, and we now know how to do this. In many ways, interventions are easier with TRA than diagnostics. Doing a full six-vessel diagnostic takes some time, similar to a transfemoral approach (TFA) diagnostic angiogram. On average, it is 3–4 minutes longer than a six-vessel TFA diagnostic. An intervention, by contrast, is just one vessel; track up the interventional catheter and you are there. Once you have the basics of catheterizing the left and right internal carotid arteries, you should

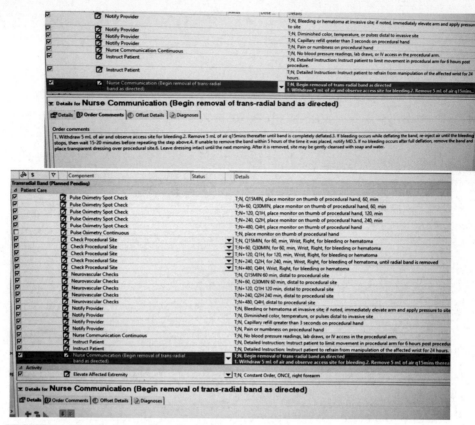

FIGURE 16.2 *Simple template of an order set.*

begin interventions. The most effective method was demonstrated by the MUSC group, whereby full and rapid conversion was employed and expertise was attained in a matter of weeks.[1]

Furthermore, one of the more common needs for TRA is in mechanical thrombectomy. As we all know, it is not uncommon for femoral access to simply not be possible, either because of severe aortic tortuosity or aorto-iliac occlusive disease (Leriche syndrome). This is not the time to be learning how to puncture the radial artery! In addition, this is not the time to be trying to get your techs to position the arm for radial access. You want your access skills and lab experience to be over the 50-case hump. If you are already adept in TRA, as well as in TRA interventions, when you see a 90-year-old headed up to your angio suite with a left M1 occlusion with a computed tomography angiogram that shows a tough arch with a bovine configuration, you should feel comfortable doing that case via TRA. If you are not confident in TRA, then you will shy away from it and flail around femorally for 45 minutes before finally going TRA and completing the case in 10 minutes. That is a disservice to the patient.

PRINCIPLE 4: DIFFERENTIATE YOURSELF WITH THE TRANSRADIAL APPROACH

Similar to all professions, there exists a spectrum of skill for operators who perform neurointervention. In addition to judgment and technical expertise, there is no question that the technique chosen impacts patient experience. When I was learning neurosurgery, there were attendings who did spinal surgeries with a huge open incision and those that did them through minimally invasive openings. For the cranial surgeries, there were attendings that shaved half of the patients head and did a huge incision and craniotomy, and there were others—for the exact same pathology—that did the procedure via a small incision and no head shave.

While they liked to argue back and forth about complications and patient outcome, the patients universally preferred the more minimally invasive techniques. It wasn't even close. As the resident seeing these patients postoperatively, there was no question that even if there was not a real "complication," the patients who had their procedure done via the less invasive option did much better with regard to pain and mobility and so on.

You should not be shy about talking to patients that you perform your procedure via TRA. There has been a huge shift toward patients becoming consumers in health care, a trend that is only going to continue. Patient comfort and preference are strong lever arms in where they seek their care, and TRA leverages these trends in a powerful way. You can drive patients to your center simply because you offer this technique.

PRINCIPLE 5: RADIAL IS A TECHNIQUE—NOT A RELIGION!

We strongly believe radial is simply a better way to undergo an endovascular procedure. The data and empirical evidence are undeniable. However, it is in the end just another tool in the armamentarium of the operator. It should be viewed as a minimally invasive neurointervention. Like all minimally invasive techniques, there are procedures where it is not the best technique. We do plenty of femoral access in our center, although it is becoming less and less common as experience grows. As industry develops radial-specific access systems, and as our experience grows, the cases that cannot be done via TRA will become less and less common. It will only get easier with time.

What is unacceptable is to simply refuse to learn the technique. To be clear, dabbling also should be considered refusal to learn TRA. You have to become adept in the technique, do at least 50 consecutive cases, and become comfortable doing the majority of diagnostic and intervention work via TRA. Then when a case comes along that you don't think makes sense to do via TRA, you are making a decision that is truly in the interests of the patient, rather than your own laziness. This is very similar to the clipping versus coiling debate that occurred when neurointervention began to take off, except it was at that time mostly between two different surgical specialities that didn't really have the ability to learn the other technique. So everyone entrenched into protectionism.

That is not the case here. All of us can easily learn TRA. We owe it to our patients to become proficient in the technique, and then make our own decision about what technique is best for each individual patient.

REFERENCE

1. Almallouhi E, Leary J, Wessell J, et al. Fast-track incorporation of the transradial approach in endovascular neurointervention. *J Neurointerv Surg.* 2020;12:176–180.

CHAPTER 17

Future Directions

AHMAD SWEID, ERIC C. PETERSON, AND PASCAL M. JABBOUR

T HE TRANSRADIAL APPROACH (TRA) WAS FIRST INTRODUCED BY CAMPEAU et al. in 1989, reporting outcomes on 100 patients undergoing diagnostic transradial angiography.[6] Building on that, Kiemeneij and Laarman employed TRA for coronary stenting. Eleven years later, in 2000, Matsumoto and colleagues described TRA for neurointerventional procedures.[14] The Radial vs. Femoral Access for Coronary Intervention (RIVAL)[11] and Radial Versus Femoral Randomized Investigation in ST-Elevation Acute Coronary Syndrome (RIFLE) showed decreased access-site morbidity in addition to mortality benefit to TRA over the transfemoral approach (TFA).[8,18] The accumulating evidence showing the superiority of the TRA compared to TFA in terms of safety, cost reductions, and patient preference culminated in a radial-first strategy recommendation by the American Heart Association. Such favorable outcomes resulted in 40% of cardiology procedures being performed through TRA. Recently, TRA has been widely embraced by neurointerventionalists.[1,7,10,12,13,15,23,25] With any new procedure or technique, perceived advantages drive the momentum for adoption, while challenges and certain limitations slow it down. The overall lag between the introduction of the transradial approach and its widespread use within the neurointerventional niche is due to a variety of factors, including perceived difficulties in navigation, lack of exposure during training, and complexity of the neurointerventional procedures.

The cardiac literature is packed with randomized clinical trials showing the safety, efficacy, and mortality benefit of TRA.[8,11,16,18,21] The superficial location of the radial artery makes it favorable to establish access and achieve hemostasis with simple compression. Its location, being confined to a tight space, decreases the risk of major complications relative to the femoral artery. There is evidence of 73% relative risk reduction in major bleeding,[10] lower rate of minor bleeding, in addition to reduced need for blood transfusions.[11] Also, there is evidence of early mobilization, shorter hospital stay, and reduced costs.[2,19] In a specific patient population, the TFA is associated with either increased risk of failure or adverse events. Elderly patients on anticoagulation, pregnant females,[22] patients with severe obesity, or patients with severe atherosclerotic disease of the ilio-femoral arteries may benefit from a TRA. Also, patients with complex vascular anatomy such as a bovine arch or aortic arch type 2 or 3 may benefit from TRA.

Despite two decades of cardiology experience and well-demonstrated safety of TRA, this approach was slowly embraced as a first-line approach by neurointerventionalists.[17] With any new technique, operators should overcome a learning curve before appreciating favorable outcomes. Extrapolating from the cardiac literature, a study of the National Cardiovascular Data Registry showed that an operator should perform 30–50 cases before reaching favorable results in terms of procedural metrics.[9,26] Similarly, a prospective randomized study by Zussman et al. showed a significant improvement in procedural efficiency with practice.[26] Multiple variables may keep operators from converting from a transfemoral to a transradial approach. The lack of training during residency (the Accreditation Council for Graduate Medical Education [ACGME] does not require residents to perform arteriography to graduate nor does it specify the approach for the arteriography), the size of the radial artery compared to the femoral artery, anatomical variants such as radioulnar loops, different set of vector forces and catheter reformation, room set-up, lack of personnel training, and lack of transradial-specific catheters.

The radial artery size is a significant limitation for TRA. Cannulating a 2.3 ± 0.4 mm is much different than cannulating a 6.6 mm femoral artery.[3,24] Failure to access the radial artery is usually due to puncture error or radial arterial spasm (RAS). These two reasons have a synergistic effect on each other, as failed attempts at piercing the radial artery result in RAS. This, in turn, results in greater difficulty in puncturing and cannulating the small artery in spasm.[5] Moreover, the ratio of the vessel caliber and the diameter of the sheath should be taken into consideration to avoid vasospasm and radial artery occlusion. The ratio should be >1 to avoid procedural limitations.[17] There are several options that can be incorporated into daily practice that have the potential to decrease the incidence of radial access failure. A double-wall puncture technique,[4] ultrasound-guided cannulation, and vasodilators can decrease the incidence of RAS. In a randomized multicenter trial, ultrasound guidance resulted in a significantly reduced number of attempts (1.65 vs. 3.0, $p <$

0.0001) and time to access (88 seconds vs. 108 seconds, $p = 0.006$), as well as improved first-pass success (64.8% vs. 43.9%, $p < 0.0001$).[21]

While neurointerventionalists have extensive experience with TFA in terms of anatomy (aortic and supra-aortic anatomy), type of catheters to use, and the vector trajectory for catheter manipulation, there are several nuts and bolts that warrant attention when performing procedures via TRA. Anatomical variations peculiar to the radial artery include radial artery loops, high brachial artery bifurcation, and accessory radial artery. Additionally, severe subclavian-innominate artery tortuosity (6%–10%) would hinder catheterizing the great vessels due to a loss of translational force because of the tortuosity, and the lack of specifically designed transradial cerebral catheters. Going more distally, arteria lusoria is an anatomical variant where the subclavian originates from the fourth aortic arch (0.6%–1.4%). Advancing the catheter through the subclavian would drop the catheter in the descending aorta.[20] Although bovine aortic arch, and type 2 and 3 aortic arches are easier to catheterize using a TRA, a type III arch creates a challenge for forming the Simmons 2 catheter in the descending or ascending aorta. The origin of the brachiocephalic artery is inferior in type 3 arch compared to type 1, which makes it more challenging to select the descending aorta. In regards to catheters, currently, there is a lack of catheters designed for TRA. The current catheters are designed for a TFA in which a vertical vector force is applied from the femoral artery to the descending aorta. Translational and rotational forces applied to the catheters are not hindered by any loops or curves, which makes it easier to select the supra-aortic vessels. While in the TRA, multiple anatomical checkpoints may hinder propagation of the forces such as navigating from the radial artery to the brachial artery, or brachial artery to the subclavian artery, or from the subclavian into the right common carotid artery. Also, it is challenging to catheterize the left vertebral artery via a right TRA with a Simmons 2 catheter. A Simmons 3 catheter with its longer distal limb makes catheterization of the left ventricle apex straightforward.[23]

Finally, work in the health system is a team effort where each personnel task is crucial for the flow of work. Training the supporting staff and educating them on the new room set-up and the positioning of the patient are paramount for success. For example, unlike the groin, the forearm and the wrist should be aligned to the level of the groin to keep catheters from falling off the table. Also, sufficient support with towels or other cushions may be placed on the extension board for the catheter platform.

The cardiac literature with its randomized clinical trials assessing every aspect of the TRA from safety, efficacy, and mortality benefit over TFA, to the radial artery puncture technique, to the use of ultrasound, to the dosing of the heparin and vasodilators sets a reliable platform for neurointerventionalists to embrace this approach.[8,11,16,18,21] However, TRA should have been adopted more quickly because of the benefits it brings to patient care. The most crucial challenge that merits focused efforts is the development of a catheter-specific TRA.

REFERENCES

1. Al Saiegh F, Mouchtouris N, Sweid A, Chalouhi N, Theofanis T, Ghosh R, et al. Placement of the Woven EndoBridge (WEB) device via distal transradial access in the anatomical snuffbox: A technical note. *J Clin Neurosci.* 2019;69:261–264.

2. Amoroso G, Sarti M, Bellucci R, Puma FL, D'Alessandro S, Limbruno U, et al. Clinical and procedural predictors of nurse workload during and after invasive coronary procedures: the potential benefit of a systematic radial access. *Eur J Cardiovasc Nurs.* 2005;4:234–241.

3. Beniwal S, Bhargava K, Kausik SK. Size of distal radial and distal ulnar arteries in adults of southern Rajasthan and their implications for percutaneous coronary interventions. *Indian Heart J.* 2014;66:506–509.

4. Bernat I, Abdelaal E, Plourde G, Bataille Y, Cech J, Pesek J, et al. Early and late outcomes after primary percutaneous coronary intervention by radial or femoral approach in patients presenting in acute ST-elevation myocardial infarction and cardiogenic shock. *Am Heart J.* 2013;165:338–343.

5. Brunet M-C, Chen SH, Peterson EC. Transradial access for neurointerventions: management of access challenges and complications. *J Neurointerv Surg.* 2020;12:82–86.

6. Campeau L. Percutaneous radial artery approach for coronary angiography. *Catheter Cardiovasc Diag.* 1989;16:3–7.

7. Chalouhi N, Sweid A, Al Saiegh F, et al. Initial Experience with Transradial Intraoperative Angiography in Aneurysm Clipping: Technique, Feasibility, and Case Series. *World Neurosurg.* 2020;134:e554–e558. doi:10.1016/j.wneu.2019.10.130

8. Hamon M, Pristipino C, Di Mario C, Nolan J, Ludwig J, Tubaro M, et al. Consensus document on the radial approach in percutaneous cardiovascular interventions: position paper by the European Association of Percutaneous Cardiovascular Interventions and Working Groups on Acute Cardiac Care and Thrombosis of the European Society of Cardiology. *EuroIntervention.* 2013;8:1242–1251.

9. Hess CN, Peterson ED, Neely ML, Dai D, Hillegass WB, Krucoff MW, et al. The learning curve for transradial percutaneous coronary intervention among operators in the United States: a study from the National Cardiovascular Data Registry. *Circulation.* 2014;129:2277–2286.

10. Jolly SS, Amlani S, Hamon M, Yusuf S, Mehta SR. Radial versus femoral access for coronary angiography or intervention and the impact on major bleeding and ischemic events: a systematic review and meta-analysis of randomized trials. *Am Heart J.* 2009;157:132–140.

11. Jolly SS, Yusuf S, Cairns J, Niemelä K, Xavier D, Widimsky P, et al. Radial versus femoral access for coronary angiography and intervention in patients with acute coronary syndromes (RIVAL): a randomised, parallel group, multicentre trial. *Lancet.* 2011;377:1409–1420.

12. Khanna O, Sweid A, Mouchtouris N, Shivashankar K, Xu V, Velagapudi L, et al. Radial artery catheterization for neuroendovascular procedures. *Stroke.* 2019;50:2587–2590.

13. Kok MM, Weernink MG, von Birgelen C, Fens A, van der Heijden LC, van Til JA. Patient preference for radial versus femoral vascular access for elective coronary procedures: the PREVAS study. *Catheter Cardiovasc Intervent.* 2018;91:17–24.

14. Matsumoto Y, Hokama M, Nagashima H, Orz Y, Toriyama T, Hongo K, et al. Transradial approach for selective cerebral angiography. *Neurol Res.* 2000;22:605–608.

15. Mouchtouris N, Al Saiegh F, Sweid A, Amllay A, Tjoumakaris S, Gooch R, et al. Transradial access for newly Food and Drug Administration–approved devices for endovascular treatment of cerebral aneurysms: a technical note. *World Neurosurg.* 2019;131:6–9.

16. Pancholy SB, Bernat I, Bertrand OF, Patel TM. Prevention of radial artery occlusion after transradial catheterization: the PROPHET-II randomized trial. *JACC: Cardiovasc Interv.* 2016;9:1992–1999.

17. Patel P, Haussen DC, Nogueira RG, Khandelwal P. The neuro radialist. *Interv Cardiol Clin.* 2020;9:75–86.

18. Romagnoli E, Biondi-Zoccai G, Sciahbasi A, Politi L, Rigattieri S, Pendenza G, et al. Radial versus femoral randomized investigation in ST-segment elevation acute coronary syndrome: the RIFLE-STEACS (Radial Versus Femoral Randomized Investigation in ST-Elevation Acute Coronary Syndrome) study. *J Am Coll Cardiol.* 2012;60:2481–2489.

19. Roussanov O, Wilson SJ, Henley K, Estacio G, Hill J, Dogan B, et al. Cost effectiveness of radial versus femoral artery approach to diagnostic cardiac catheterization. *J Inv Cardiol.* 2007;19:349.

20. Scala C, Leone Roberti Maggiore U, Candiani M, Venturini P, Ferrero S, Greco T, et al. Aberrant right subclavian artery in fetuses with Down syndrome: a systematic review and meta-analysis. *Ultrasound Obstet Gynecol.* 2015;46:266–276.

21. Seto AH, Roberts JS, Abu-Fadel MS, Czak SJ, Latif F, Jain SP, et al. Real-time ultrasound guidance facilitates transradial access: RAUST (Radial Artery access with Ultrasound Trial). *JACC: Cardiovasc Interv.* 2015;8:283–291.

22. Shah SS, Snelling BM, Brunet MC, Sur S, McCarthy DJ, Stein A, et al. Transradial mechanical thrombectomy for proximal middle cerebral artery occlusion in a first trimester pregnancy: case report and literature review. *World Neurosurg.* 2018;120:415–419.

23. Snelling BM, Sur S, Shah SS, Khandelwal P, Caplan J, Haniff R, et al. Transradial cerebral angiography: techniques and outcomes. *J Neurointerv Surg.* 2018;10:874–881.

24. Spector KS, Lawson WE. Optimizing safe femoral access during cardiac catheterization. *Catheter Cardiovasc Intervent.* 2001;53:209–212.

25. Sweid A, Starke RM, Herial N, Chalouhi N, Xu V, Shivashankar K, et al. Transradial approach for the treatment of brain aneurysms using flow diversion: feasibility, safety, and outcomes. *J Neurosurg Sci.* 2019;63:509–517.

26. Zussman BM, Tonetti DA, Stone J, Brown M, Desai SM, Gross BA, et al. Maturing institutional experience with the transradial approach for diagnostic cerebral arteriography: overcoming the learning curve. *J Neurointerv Surg.* 2019;11:1235–1238.

Index

For the benefit of digital users, indexed terms that span two pages (e.g., 52–53) may, on occasion, appear on only one of those pages.

Figures and tables are indicated by *f* and *t* following the page number.